T0073408

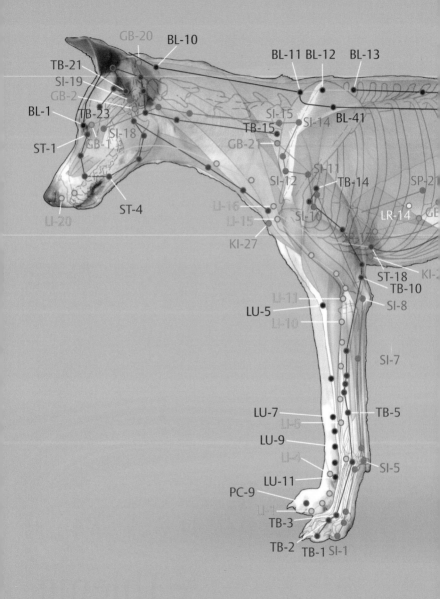

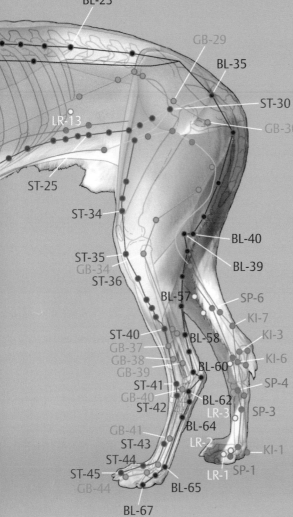

BL-23

GB-29

BL-35

ST-30

GB-30

LR-13

ST-25

ST-34

BL-40

BL-39

ST-35

GB-34

ST-36

BL-57

SP-6

KI-7

ST-40

BL-58

KI-3

GB-37

KI-6

GB-38

GB-39

BL-60

SP-4

ST-41

GB-40

BL-62

SP-3

ST-42

LR-3

GB-41

BL-64

ST-43

LR-2

KI-1

ST-44

BL-65

LR-1

SP-1

ST-45

GB-44

BL-67

Acupuncture for Dogs and Cats

A Pocket Atlas

Second Edition

Christina Eul-Matern, DVM
IVAS Certified Veterinary Acupuncturist (CVA)
VetSensus Mastertherapist (VSCETAO)
ICREO Authorization for Further Training in Acupuncture from the Veterinary
Chamber of Hessen, Germany;
Head of VetSensus Institute for Sensological Diagnostics and Therapy
and Tiergesundheitszentrum Idstein (TGZ)
Idstein, Germany

207 illustrations

Thieme
Stuttgart • New York • Delhi • Rio de Janeiro

Library of Congress Cataloging-in-Publication Data is available with the publisher.

This book is an authorized translation of the 3rd German edition published and copyrighted 2018 by Sonntag Verlag in Georg Thieme Verlag, Stuttgart. Title of the German edition: Taschenatlas Akupunktur bei Hund und Katze

Translator: Sabine Wilms, PhD, Langley/WA, USA

Drawings:
Templates: Martina Steinmetz, Dielkirchen, Germany; Dana Müller, Maintal, Germany
Executed by: Malgorzata and Piotr Gusta, Paris, France; Angelika Brauner, Hohengeißenberg, Germany

Georg Thieme Verlag KG
Rüdigerstrasse 14, 70469 Stuttgart, Germany
+49 [0]711 8931 421, customerservice@thieme.de

Cover design: © Thieme.
Cover illustration:
Template: Martina Steinmetz, Dielkirchen, Germany
Executed by: Malgorzata and Piotr Gusta, Paris, France

Typesetting by DiTech Process Solutions, India

Printed in Germany by Beltz Grafische Betriebe
5 4 3 2 1

ISBN 978-3-13-243454-7

Also available as an e-book:
eISBN (PDF): 978-3-13-243455-4
eISBN (epub): 978-3-13-257915-6

Important note: Medicine is an ever-changing science undergoing continual development. Research and clinical experience are continually expanding our knowledge, in particular our knowledge of proper treatment and drug therapy. Insofar as this book mentions any dosage or application, readers may rest assured that the authors, editors, and publishers have made every effort to ensure that such references are in accordance with **the state of knowledge at the time of production of the book.**

Nevertheless, this does not involve, imply, or express any guarantee or responsibility on the part of the publishers in respect to any dosage instructions and forms of applications stated in the book. **Every user is requested to examine carefully** the manufacturers' leaflets accompanying each drug and to check, if necessary in consultation with a physician or specialist, whether the dosage schedules mentioned therein or the contraindications stated by the manufacturers differ from the statements made in the present book. Such examination is particularly important with drugs that are either rarely used or have been newly released on the market. Every dosage schedule or every form of application used is entirely at the user's own risk and responsibility. The authors and publishers request every user to report to the publishers any discrepancies or inaccuracies noticed. If errors in this work are found after publication, errata will be posted at www.thieme.com on the product description page.

Some of the product names, patents, and registered designs referred to in this book are in fact registered trademarks or proprietary names even though specific reference to this fact is not always made in the text. Therefore, the appearance of a name without designation as proprietary is not to be construed as a representation by the publisher that it is in the public domain.

Thieme addresses people of all gender identities equally. We encourage our authors to use gender-neutral or gender-equal expressions wherever the context allows.

FSC
www.fsc.org
MIX
Papier aus verantwortungsvollen Quellen
FSC® C089473

Contents

Foreword

I first met Dr. Christina Eul-Matern at a meeting of the German Society for Holistic Veterinary Medicine (Gesellschaft für Ganzheitliche Tiermedizin; GGTM) in Nuremberg in 2006. At that time, she was working with other colleagues to form the German IVAS Affiliate (GERVAS). I was impressed not only by her knowledge of acupuncture but also by her dedication in forming an organization that would provide acupuncturists in Germany with another avenue to meet and join forces in the promotion of acupuncture and Chinese medicine. Through her efforts and those of her colleagues, GERVAS is a young but strong and enthusiastic organization. She was also committed in providing a solid education of Traditional Chinese Veterinary Medicine (TCVM) and acupuncture to veterinarians and saw the IVAS-based curriculum model as ideal to teach veterinarians about TCVM and acupuncture in an organized, concise, and efficient manner, allowing veterinarians to complete the training within a year.

Dr. Eul-Matern remains committed to teaching and disseminating important information about acupuncture and TCVM, as evidenced by this atlas. *Acupuncture for Dogs and Cats* is well written, giving a concise but accurate review of TCVM and the bones of Chinese medical philosophy. Included in the first section are synopses of the Fundamental Substances, the *zang fu* organs—their relations to each other and their functions, primarily in accordance with the Five Element theory—and the various channel systems of the body. The author has distilled some of the most pertinent information regarding the Chinese understanding of medical physiology and has presented it in an easy-to-understand

and relevant format. The TCVM diagnostics section is brief and to the point, again providing veterinarians new to the world of acupuncture with a handy "go-to" reference section to understand the various diagnostic methods and paradigms that exist in TCVM. Interspersed between the text are well-presented drawings and tables that assist the reader in understanding basic and important concepts.

The second half of the first section of the book focuses on the acupuncture points that are most commonly used in animals today. Again, the author has successfully distilled the important characteristics and categories of points and their functions, beginning with an overview of various groupings of points and their functions and indications. The clear drawings accompanying this section of the book, which illustrate the location of these groups of points in relation to each other, are a very useful learning aid. The accompanying tables provide a quick and easy reference for veterinarians trying to categorize all of the new information regarding acupuncture.

The majority of the book focuses on the acupuncture points that are used in animals—their functions, locations, indications, and advice on needling techniques. Even the Chinese names and characters are given, something I have a personal interest in. What I find particularly useful about this atlas is that all the points on each of the channels are described. These include all of the transpositional points as well as some of the traditional points. The illustrations that accompany the point descriptions are impressive—not just in their quality but in showing the described points in relation to other nearby points. This is a great learning aid not only for new practitioners of veterinary acupuncture but also as a reminder for those of us with more experience.

It has been a pleasure to meet Christina and work with her on a limited basis, and I am honored that she asked me to write a foreword for her book. I had seen the atlas during courses in Germany and was disappointed that it was only available in German. Now this much-needed, concise reference book is also available in English and I would recommend it to any veterinarians learning acupuncture as well as to those with some experience. It will be a benefit to any veterinarian for years as they strive to understand all of the nuances of Chinese medical theory and how to use acupuncture to help our four-legged friends.

Linda Boggie, DVM
IVAS Certified Veterinary Acupuncturist
The Netherlands

Preface to the Second English Edition

Because emotional factors are also highly relevant for illness in animals, I have decided to expand the third German edition of this book by incorporating the psychological effects of acupuncture points. Furthermore, I have added a chapter on the five elements and their connection to the psyche. This is intended to take into account an important aspect of animal acupuncture.

I want to take the opportunity here to thank Dana Müller who, as part of her acupuncture training, took all the illustrations to create a comprehensive chart for the cover pages, to offer a quick overview to the reader.

Christina Eul-Matern, DVM

Preface to the First English Edition

When a friend introduced me to Chinese medicine many years ago, my attitude toward holistic therapies changed rapidly. I had been conscious of the limited options for disease prevention in biomedicine for a long time and now seemed to have finally found a way to recognize health-related imbalances early on and even to avert disorders altogether. Countless scientific studies were able to substantiate this fact. For me as a veterinarian with a doctorate in Western veterinary medicine, this was great news. Research on topics such as the stimulation of vasoactive substances like serotonin, adrenaline, and endorphins or the effects of acupuncture on the autonomous nervous system aroused my interest.

Already during my training and even more so after years of clinical experience, after I began my activity as lecturer on animal acupuncture, discussions broke out again and again on therapies as well as point localizations. In this context it is important to know that in contrast to today, acupuncture in early China did not know of the exact point descriptions. At that time, it would be more accurate to speak of reactive areas than precise points. Even today, acupuncturists are still well advised to test the reactivity of an acupuncture point at the described location before needling it. To touch, palpate, and feel where the correct point is located, that is and remains an important aspect of acupuncture. The discussion on exact localizations is also kept alive by the fact that contemporary animal acupuncture in the West uses the two systems of transposed and traditional points side by side. Taking into consideration the physical changes in the course of evolution, the practice of transposing point localizations from the human body to the animal also contains a certain potential for variations.

Animal acupuncture is increasingly being integrated into our Western healthcare system and scientifically examined and developed. Specialists all over the world are studying the effect, origin, and exact localization of individual points and exchanging their findings. The present work is an attempt to bring together all current information and tie it into a single atlas fit for the clinic. I have compared relevant information from the leading educational organizations and educators of animal acupuncture with the experiences from my own practice and taken this as a basis. This approach was utilized both for point localizations as well as for their effect and indications. In addition, for the effect and indications of acupuncture points, I have also taken into consideration the practical and Western-scientific experiences of modern animal acupuncturists.

Among all the possible justifications for the efficacy of acupuncture, however, one point is of particular importance to me: Acupuncture is an energy-based system of healing. All university education and long years of training in Chinese medicine do not change the fact that we bring our own energies into play when we practice acupuncture.

The literature on Chinese medicine contains numerous allusions to this factor: Needling techniques explain how we bring more or less *qi* into the organism or pull it out by changing the direction in which we twist the needle or the speed during insertion. Hand position (e.g., middle finger on HT-8) during needling is also meant to protect the practitioner's own *qi*.

Good posture and attitude during needling are said to stabilize the practitioner and optimize treatment results. More than anything, though, a necessary prerequisite for any successful treatment is mutual trust, openness, and the willingness to help or be helped. I, therefore, appeal to anyone engaged in Chinese medicine and acupuncture to be attentive to the processes that take place on an energetic level and, if necessary, to continue training also in this area.

Now that Thieme Publishers has translated the pocket atlas *Acupuncture for Dogs and Cats* into English so soon after its German publication, I am overjoyed that this text will reach the international community of veterinarians and animal acupuncturists. I look forward to constructive pointers and collaboration.

Christina Eul-Matern, DVM

Acknowledgments

Here I want to express my gratitude to those without whose support this work would have never been possible in the first place, as well as to those who took charge so energetically of the English translation.

First of all, my thanks go to my students who pointed out again and again with matchless persistence the necessity of composing this atlas, thereby giving me the necessary motivation. Your ideas and suggestions were very useful.

Next, I want to thank my colleagues Dr. Brigitte Traenckner and Dr. Jean Yves Guray for having infected me with their enthusiasm for Chinese veterinary medicine and for giving me numerous new impulses, especially in the initial stages, which greatly accelerated my path.

I thank Christine Kinbach for her constructive suggestions for this book and for her consistent support, which has helped me along again and again.

In addition, special thanks go to my colleague Dr. Martina Steinmetz, who contributed greatly to the success of this book with her wonderful drawings, and to Suse Capelle, whose creativity has already helped me in so many ways. Her photographs of dogs and cats have become part of the foundations for this atlas.

I also want to thank Leon, our Podenco, for his patient collaboration and our kitty Smilla for her voluntary posing.

You have done a fantastic job!

My dear family members, Hans-Karl, Anika, and Carina, deserve my deepest gratitude as well. They supported me and always granted me the space to work on this book in important moments.

I thank my parents who have always believed in me and have given me the feeling that everything that is truly important is within my reach.

Lastly, I thank Angelika Findgott and Anne Lamparter from Thieme Publishers, who have produced and optimized this wonderful translated edition with exceptional dedication and professionalism. For the translation itself, though, I have to thank Dr. Sabine Wilms. In an unparalleled manner, she has worked through, supplemented, and translated my writings, tables, and illustrations.

My heartfelt thanks to all of you!

Christina Eul-Matern, DVM

Note from the Translator

It is a rare treat for a translator to be involved in a project with as much personal appeal and connections as I have enjoyed in the present book. As a farmer and animal lover myself, I have been so happy to find Dr. Matern's empathetic concern and experience in caring for our four-legged friends expressed on every page. As a lecturer and author on classical Chinese medicine for humans, I have found her clinical insights inspiring and her distinctly personal perspective refreshing, and I have been fascinated by her skillful integration of the traditional concepts of Chinese medicine with her clinical experience and modern scientific research. In my mind, the contents of this book and Dr. Matern's style of veterinary medicine ultimately reflect the author's understanding of the connections between humans and animals and the macrocosm at large.

It has been an honor to play a small part in bringing this book to the larger audience it deserves. My only hope is that the clinical advice contained herein will find abundant application, to the benefit of all the cats and dogs out there!

Sabine Wilms, PhD

I Basic Concepts of Acupuncture

1 What Does Acupuncture Have to Offer?

Acupuncture is an energy-based system of healing that is several thousand years old and addresses and activates the self-healing powers of the body. Biomedicine therefore classifies it as a form of "regulatory medicine."

The stimulation of acupuncture points influences the flow of energy within the body along the channels and hence in the entire organism. Acupuncture resolves blockages, moves stagnations, supplies emptiness with new energy, and relieves fullness. As a result, pain can be reduced and disturbed organ functions can be revived. Successful acupuncture restores the natural balance of the organism. It is not able, however, to heal permanently destroyed tissue.

One important aspect of this healing process is that the body learns through acupuncture to restore its balance on its own. The acupuncturist thereby has the role of showing the diseased organism the path to healing by means of the needle. Ideally, if identical problems reappear later, the patient's self-healing powers will "remember" this path and start functioning on their own in the way that they have learned earlier.

During acupuncture treatment, fine needles are inserted at precisely localized acupuncture points and retained there for a certain amount of time. The length of time that the needles remain in the body depends on the indication and condition of the patient. To avoid injury to the underlying tissue and to nerves, blood vessels, joints, or organs, this treatment should only be performed by trained and qualified practitioners.

Animal acupuncture originally worked with individual, empirically discovered points and their combinations. A system of channels did not exist. This was only developed later, resulting in the systematization of animal acupuncture. This led to the development of the so-called **"transposed system"** of animal acupuncture, which differs from the classical points especially in the location of the back *shu* points. In the process of transposing, the location of these diagnostically and therapeutically useful acupuncture points was transferred from their location in the human body to their location in animals. The system was then refined further, primarily by medical doctors and later also by veterinarians. In clinical practice, veterinarians often supplement the transposed system with classical points of Traditional Chinese Veterinary Medicine (TCVM).

For the following disorders, TCVM and acupuncture can have a helpful or at least a supportive effect:

- Movement disorders; for example, due to arthrosis or arthritis in the hip, shoulder, elbow, knee, spinal column, and toes
- Growth and development disorders of the bones and joints
- Geriatric problems
- Chronic disorders of the respiratory tract, skin, gastrointestinal tract, urogenital tract, cardiovascular system, eyes, and ears
- Allergies and disorders of the immune system
- Hormonal disturbances, as in diabetes mellitus, Cushing's disease, thyroid problems, ovarian cysts, and fertility disorders
- Epilepsy
- Tumors
- Psychological problems, such as pathological fears, aggression, etc.

At the same time, acupuncture can reduce the dosages of pharmaceutical drugs that may be necessary.

In all of these cases, the basic requirements for a successful treatment are a thorough medical history, examination, and diagnosis. The mere application of standardized needling formulas without knowledge of their background carries the risk of exacerbating the disorder and carrying it deeper into the body instead of improving or to say nothing of healing it.

The complex system of Chinese medicine was developed over several thousand years, partly on the basis of observations and experiences gathered and documented by individual practitioners. Over a long period of time, a large number of patients provided huge amounts of informative data. The evaluation of this material made it possible to discern general patterns that finally gave rise to a coherent medical philosophy. This philosophy aims at preserving the health of the individual by means of controlling and balancing actions on the inside and outside. Our Western knowledge of Chinese medicine and acupuncture is built on this groundwork, allowing for a well-informed application of acupuncture.

In my research, I have come across the following statement several times. I find it very meaningful and would therefore like to share it with you. The statement is from the preface of the extensively studied and often-cited classic *Qian Jin Yao Fang (Essential Formulas Worth a Thousand Pieces of Gold)* in which Sun Simiao (a Tang dynasty physician) describes the preparations required for anyone who wants to study medicine:

- "First, you must familiarize yourself with the *Su Wen* (*Plain Questions*), *Jia Yi Jing* (*A-Z Classic of Acupuncture and Moxibustion*), and *Huang Di Nei Jing* (*Inner Classic of the Yellow Emperor*) (three classic texts of Chinese medicine), the 12 channels, the Chinese pulse locations, the five viscera and six bowels (the internal 'organs' of Chinese medicine), the inside, the outside, the points, the medicinals, and the classic formulas.
- Additionally, you must understand *yin* and *yang* and acquire the ability to recognize life's fortune (to read a person's destiny from their face), to use the *Yi Jing* (*Classic of Changes*) (fortune-telling).
- You must know the meaning of justice, humaneness, and virtue. As well as compassion, sorrow, luck, and giving. You must also study the five phases of change as well as geography and astronomy ..."

These realizations are 1300 years old and still hold true today. Well-founded knowledge, life experience, and insight into human nature are indispensable for the correct evaluation of any state of health. Empathy, the desire to help, openness, and the willingness to give love are prerequisites for healing.

2 History of Acupuncture

To convey an impression of the time frame for the development of veterinary acupuncture, the following section lists some benchmarks:

In the **Shang dynasty** (1766–122 BCE), veterinary knowledge was documented for the first time. Inscriptions on bones describe disorders of both humans and animals. "Horse priests" used their healing powers to treat horses. One of their methods was the early use of the precursor of the modern *Yi Jing* (*Classic of Changes*). For this oracle, animal bones or turtle shells were heated and then interpreted by reading the resulting cracks.

During the **Zhou dynasty**/Chou dynasty (11th century to 476 BCE), the theory of *yin* and *yang* and that of the five elements was established. In this period, a large amount of veterinary knowledge was documented. As recorded in the historical text *Zhou Li Tian Guan* (*History of the Zhou Dynasty*), there were already full-time professional veterinarians. Another book from this time, the *Li Ji* (*Book of Rites*) describes the collection of medicinal herbs and also some serious animal diseases. The first veterinarian referred to by name was Chao Fu. The *Huang Di Nei Jing* (*Inner Classic of the Yellow Emperor*), which was composed in the Warring States period, states that acupuncture developed in Southern China, moxibustion in Northern China, medicinal therapy in Western China, and massage and acupressure in Central China. In this period, there were veterinarians who specialized in the treatment of equine disorders. Some of these books described various disorders of domestic animals. The needles used for acupuncture were made of iron.

During the **Qin dynasty**/Ch'in dynasty (221–209 BCE), the government issued laws governing livestock breeding and

veterinary medicine, which is documented in the text *Jiu* (*Yuan*) *Lu* (*Livestock Breeding and Rules of Veterinary Medicine*).

In 1930, archaeologists discovered slips of bamboo in the desert of Western China that date from the **Han dynasty** (206 BCE to 220 CE) and contain formulas of medicinal therapy for animals. Some books from the time of Zhang Zhongjing (Zhang Ji) (about 150–219 CE) describe animal treatments that combine acupuncture and pharmacotherapy. There were also veterinarians specializing in cattle.

Around 500 CE, a training center and agency for veterinary medicine were established. Different books on veterinary medicine were composed.

During the **Sui dynasty** (581–618 CE), a government agency for veterinary medicine and livestock breeding (Tai Pu Si) was set up, subsequently employing 120 veterinarians. Several books were published on equine medicine, among them an atlas for channels and acupuncture for horses.

During the **Tang dynasty** (618–907 CE), a comprehensive educational system for veterinary medicine was established. Between 705 and 707 CE, there were 600 veterinarians, four teachers, and 100 students at the Tai Pu Si. The *Si Mu An Ji Ji* (*Collection of Ways to Care for and Treat Horses*) is a book that systematically presents basic knowledge, diagnosis, and therapeutic techniques of Chinese veterinary medicine. In 659 CE, the government published the *Xin Xiu Ben Cao* (*Newly Revised Materia Medica*), which described 844 Chinese medicinal herbs for humans and animals.

During the **Song dynasty** (960–1279 CE), Bing Ma Jian opened its doors as the first hospital for horses. They had so much work to do there that a plea went out in 1036 to consult other establishments for less serious cases. The famous veterinarian Chang Shun lived during this time.

In the **Yuan dynasty** (1279–1368 CE), Bian Bao wrote his famous book *Ji Tong Xuan Lun* (*Treatment of Sick Horses*).

During the **Ming dynasty** (1368–1644 CE), every owner of more than 25 horses had to provide two or three young men for the study of veterinary medicine. Many famous books on veterinary medicine were composed. Probably the most famous of these is the *Liao Ma Ji* (*The Treatment of Horses*), which was written by the Yü brothers after 60 years of clinical experience.

In the period from the **Qing dynasty/** Ching dynasty to the Opium War (1644–1840 CE), veterinary medicine developed little in China. We know of a few books on cattle diseases. In 1683, the German physician Dr. E. Kampfer (as did some French merchants at the same time) brought acupuncture to Europe.

Entering the **Modern Age** (1840–1949 CE), China had no interest in TCVM. Nevertheless, veterinarians kept it alive in their practice. Only two known books survive from this period—one on many types of animals including dogs and cats by Li Nanhui, and a unique book from 1900 on swine diseases, *Zhu Jin Da Quan* (*Complete Collection of Swine Diseases*), which contains 63 examples of complete formulas.

Western veterinary medicine (WVM) reached China at the beginning of the 20th century. A private school for WVM was opened in Shanghai.

Recent developments (1949 to present): The People's Republic of China under Mao Zedong attempted to revive and develop TCVM and issued an edict on this matter in 1956. In the same year, the first National Congress for Popular Veterinary Medicine was held in Beijing. Here, participants were urged to combine Traditional Chinese with conventional Western medicine, in order to join the respective advantages of each system and to allow them to support each other.

Each therapy has its strengths and weaknesses. TCVM can treat disorders and thereby reduce sensitivity to certain disturbances. WVM has advanced diagnostic possibilities that can directly reveal the cause of a disease and pathogens. TCVM directs its attention to restoring the balance in the whole body so that it is better able to face stress factors and maintain its health. WVM addresses pathological symptoms and searches for causes in the form of agents, tissue injuries, dysfunctions, etc.

In the People's Republic of China, training and research centers for TCVM were once again established. The publication of acupuncture analgesia has had a breakthrough effect, impressing Chinese and Western experts equally. New acupuncture techniques and formulas have been developed and as a result attention to acupuncture has grown tremendously since 1978.

Oswald Kothbauer from Grieskirchen in Austria was one of the first practicing Western veterinarians to apply acupuncture. He has written several scientific treatises on the subject of animal acupuncture and has thereby contributed to the development of this field in the West. Kothbauer was the first Western scientist who managed to perform acupuncture analgesia on a cow, the results of which he published in 1973.

Since the founding of the International Veterinary Acupuncture Society (IVAS) in the United States in 1974, veterinary acupuncture has developed rapidly all over the world, not least because of the founding of numerous affiliated national organizations.

In 2004, with the help of engaged colleagues the author was able to establish the first association of pure acupuncture veterinarians in Germany, the German Veterinary Acupuncture Society (GERVAS). Its objective is to promote the spread and quality assurance of veterinary acupuncture by means of qualified training and collegial exchange.

Today, we stimulate acupuncture points by a variety of methods. Different needles (steel, gold, silver, and platinum) are used (see Chapter 10, Acupuncture Needles (p.60)), and laser, ultrasound, crystal, magnetic acupuncture, and moxibustion are examples of modern techniques in animal acupuncture (see Chapter 10, Alternatives to Needle Acupuncture (p.62)). Acupuncture is known all over the world and has established itself in many countries. Veterinary universities and especially volunteer-led veterinary organizations have been engaged intensively in the development and training of Chinese animal acupuncture and medicinal therapy. The nonprofit organizations that currently offer state-certified training for veterinarians are the IVAS in the USA, Norwegian Acupuncture Society (NoVAS) in Norway, and the Akademie für Tierärztliche Fortbildung/ Gesellschaft für Ganzheitliche Tiermedizin (ATF/GGTM) and GERVAS in Germany.

From 2016 to 2019, the author has been able to follow her colleague Detlef Rittmann in offering acupuncture/osteopathy as an elective to students in the School of Veterinary Medicine at the Justus-Liebig-Universität in Gießen, with an overwhelming response. The author is also teaching animal acupuncture as a lecturer at the Fresenius University of Applied Sciences in Idstein. Hopefully, these appointments are only a beginning and an important step for the acceptance of Chinese medicine. Individual veterinarians and alternative veterinary practitioners are also working successfully in this area. In order to promote the development of veterinary acupuncture and energetic veterinary medicine in this complex situation to the best of her abilities, the author decided in 2013 to establish a separate educational institute called VetSensus.

3 The Principles of Traditional Chinese Medicine

3.1 Difference between Western Medicine and TCM

While Western medicine focuses on detecting and eliminating the cause of a disorder, Eastern medicine sees the origin of disease in the interaction of various, mutually interdependent internal and external influences. The Chinese physician looks for the threads that connect individual processes in the organism and merges them into one common effect. This is the point at which he or she recognizes nonphysiological patterns and shows the body the way back into healthy channels. Misdirected energies are steered back in the right direction, and the body is shown the way to self-healing.

In Traditional Chinese Medicine (TCM), the underlying goal is to integrate all the potential variables of a disorder into the patient's clinical picture and include them in the treatment. This approach entails a direct contradiction to current research and treatment methods of Western medicine, whose goal is to control and, if possible, eliminate all variables. In individual cases, a deviation of symptoms from the norm can lead to problems with diagnosis or treatment.

Western medicine tends to analyze individual symptoms to understand the cause of a disorder. For this purpose, it has developed sophisticated diagnostic systems such as imaging techniques and laboratory diagnostics.

3.2 Important Terms in TCM

3.2.1 The Basic Substances

The five basic substances are:
- *Qi* (life energy)
- *Xue* (blood)
- *Jing* (essence)
- *Shen* (vital spirit)
- *Jin ye* (bodily fluids)

Qi

From the philosophical or cosmological perspective, *qi* is the true source of the entire universe and of life in general. It is the basic substance of which the world and hence also the human body is composed. It is only as the result of the tension between *yin* and *yang* that this activating energy in our world is created.

The body's own *qi* moves the organism and, depending on its function, has different characteristics. To begin with, each organ and each functional cycle have their own *qi* with the specific characteristics required in that context.

In general, the functions of *qi* are:
- Moving
- Protecting
- Transforming
- Preserving
- Warming

In addition, there are different manifestations of *qi* in the body, which fulfill a variety of functions.

Zong Qi The respiratory or gathering *qi* is connected to the heart and lung. It gathers in the thorax and directs the rhythm of the breath.

Yuan Qi The source *qi* is the refined, energetic form of essence and has its source in the kidneys. It circulates in the body and activates all organs. It gathers in the *yuan* source points and courses through the triple burner.

Gu Qi The food *qi* is formed from ingested food by the spleen and then ascends into the thorax. There, it is transformed into blood in the heart and, in combination with air, forms the *zong qi* in the lung.

Zhen Qi The true *qi* is the last stage of refined *qi* and has two manifestations: *wei qi* and *ying qi*.

Wei Qi One aspect of *qi* which defends the body. It is the external protection (defense *qi*). *Wei qi* courses closely underneath the skin and regulates the sweat glands.

Ying Qi This is the nutritive *qi* that is linked to the blood (*xue*) and assists in transforming the purest nutrients into blood. *Xue* and *ying* are inseparable. "Battalion, barrack, camp, operational, searching" are translations for this term. All these terms are in the widest sense related to the notion of provisioning. *Ying* extracts itself and becomes blood. It nourishes the viscera and moistens the bowels. It originates from food (nutrients).

Xue

Xue is equated with blood. It is the material aspect of *qi*.

Jing

Jing (essence) is the earth aspect of the three treasures *shen*, *qi*, and *jing*, and thereby carries the greatest *yin* energy. *Jing* stands for the inherited substance/DNA and is an internally produced substance that should be preserved. Earlier heaven essence (*xian tian zhi jing*) is bestowed already on the fetus during conception and is very difficult to reproduce. It is consumed in the course of one's life.

Later heaven essence (*hou tian zhi jing*) can be replaced daily by the spleen and stomach with a healthy diet.

Shen

Shen is the spirit, consciousness, vitality, or external manifestation of the internal condition of the body. Thinking is the dominant aspect of this concept. *Shen* manifests in the memory and in sleep, emanates from the eyes, and means "wonderful," "mysterious," and is related to the eternal dimension of life, to the magical and heavenly aspects of being alive. *Shen* is the *yang* aspect of the three treasures *shen*, *qi*, and *jing*. It connects us to heaven and brings us our *dao*.

Jin Ye

Jin ye are all the other fluids except for blood (*xue*). They are two completely different substances: *Jin* is a thin fluid that nourishes the skin and muscles and enters the blood. It forms sweat and urine. *Ye* is the thicker part that nourishes the bones, internal organs, brain, and marrow. It moistens openings and joints. Both of these come from the essence of our food.

3.2.2 Zang Fu

Zang fu is the Chinese term for the internal organs (▶ Table 3.1). *Zang* are the visceral or storage organs. *Fu* are the bowels or hollow organs, which have the role of collecting and eliminating. The viscera and bowels are linked to the 12 main channels.

Table 3.1 Viscera and bowels

Viscera (*yin*)	Bowels (*yang*)
Liver	Gallbladder
Heart	Small intestine
Pericardium	Triple burner
Spleen	Stomach
Lung	Large intestine
Kidney	Bladder

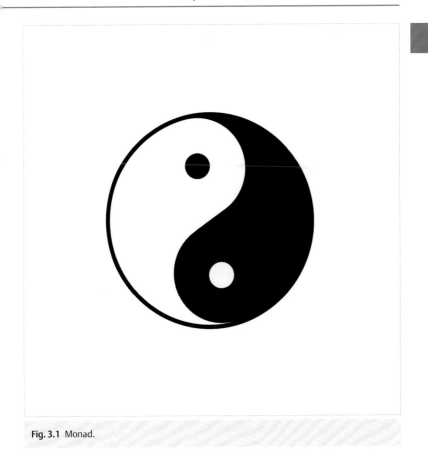

Fig. 3.1 Monad.

3.2.3 *Yin* and *Yang*

❗ *Yin* and *yang* are complementary opposites that form the basis of all phenomena and events in the universe. They are a developmental stage in the cosmological sequence.

Life means transformation. The monad *tai ji* (▶ Fig. 3.1) symbolizes the relationship between *yin* and *yang*. The lower, black section of the circle symbolizes *yin* within *yin*, while the upper, white section stands for *yang* within *yang*. Both halves continuously change into each other and carry the seed of the other in them. We can see the polarity of *yin* and *yang* in animate and inanimate nature as well as in every living creature (▶ Fig. 3.2).

Originally, *yin* and *yang* were compared with the properties of the two sides of a

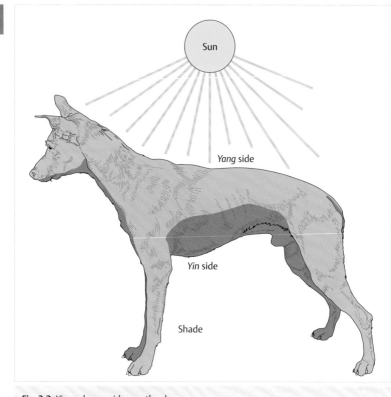

Fig. 3.2 *Yin* and *yang* sides on the dog.

mountain. The darker, cooler, lower side corresponded to *yin*; the brighter, warmer, upper side to *yang*. Consequently, *yin* was also associated with the sinking of fog, the condensation of water, slowness, stillness, gathering and containing, the inside, heaviness, depth, nurturing, the feminine, and the night. *Yang,* on the other hand, referred to warmth, dispersing, evaporation, activity, movement, speed, the outside, pushing, the masculine, and the day.

Heaven (seat of the sun) is *yang*; the earth is *yin.*

Functions of *Yang*

- Source of warmth
- Moving
- Securing
- Protecting
- Transforming

Functions of *Yin*

- Cooling
- Moistening
- Nourishing
- Transmitting stillness

The **four principles** of *yin* and *yang* are:
1. *Yin* and *yang* constitute opposites and contain each other's seeds in them.
2. *Yin* and *yang* can change into each other.
3. *Yin* and *yang* are mutually dependent.
4. *Yin* and *yang* consume and control each other.

It is impossible for *yin* and *yang* to exist on their own. Without light, there can be no shade; without mountain, no valley; without cold, no warmth.

The harmonious balance of *yin* and *yang* is essential for the healthy function of body and soul.

Opposites do not exclude each other—they need each other. A wonderful image for this relationship is the magnetic rod, which always has a north and a south pole, regardless of how often you cut and divide it.

3.2.4 The Five Elements (Phases of Change)

There are five phases (*wu xing*) which are each associated with one element (water, wood, fire, earth, and metal). The phases of change refer to the material world and the relationship of different substances to each other (▶ Table 3.2).

Water

The governing energy of water is cold. Winter with its inwardly directed energy is associated with it. Slowed-down processes and movements embody passivity, rigidity, and hardness. Bones and teeth belong here. The emotion of fear also leads to rigidity. Deep water is black and salty; the smell is putrid. The kidney and bladder are associated with water. Cold triggers the urge to urinate. Cold feet can at first harm the bladder and kidney. Cold-induced pain is strictly localized, gnawing, and persistent. The ear, conveniently shaped like a kidney, is the sensory organ at which the kidney opens.

Well-known expressions that can serve as mnemonic aids are:
- "We are scared to the bone."
- "I am scared stiff."
- "It sends cold shivers up and down the spine."
- "To wet one's pants [in fear]."

Wood

The association here is with the dynamic properties of wind. The green color of a windy spring, sour taste, and rancid smell are also related to wood. Excessive anger injures the liver. Damage can often be seen in discolored sclera. Rage makes irate eyes appear reddish, tenses muscles, and causes them to remain tense. The mobility of the muscles, tendons, and the most mobile sensory organ of the body, that is, the eye, with its numerous muscles, are associated with it (pure muscle mass, however, is related to the earth phase). Correlated organs are the liver and gallbladder.

Wind disorders are marked by sudden changes. They can be caused by exposure to wind and drafts, leading to symptoms like lumbago and stiff neck, but they can also be due to internal causes and then lead to, for example, epilepsy, migraines, itching, and apoplexy.

Wind is the vehicle by which all pathological factors can more easily penetrate into the body. It is not rare for alcoholics, for example, to have disturbed aggressive behavior.

Some expressions that can serve as mnemonic aids are:
- "It makes the bile rise in my throat."
- "His response was full of bile and hatred."

Fire

The key notion here is heat not only as an environmental influence, but also as an

Table 3.2 Correlations with the phases

	Water	Wood	Fire	Earth	Metal
Season	Winter	Spring	Summer	Late summer	Autumn
Climate	Cold	Wind	Heat	Dampness	Dryness
Sensory organ	Ears	Eyes	Tongue	Mouth	Nose
Smell	Putrid	Rancid-pungent	Burnt	Aromatic	Musty
Flavor	Salty	Sour	Burnt, bitter	Sweet	Hot-spicy
Harmful emotion	Fear/panic	Rage/irritation	Joy/hectic	Brooding/prejudice	Sadness/dissociation
Color	Black	Green	Red	Yellow	White
Viscus (*yin*)	Kidney	Liver	Heart/pericardium	Spleen	Lung
Bowel (*yang*)	Bladder	Gallbladder	Triple burner, small intestine	Stomach	Large intestine
Tissue	Bones, teeth	Tendons, ligaments	Blood vessels	Muscles, connective tissue	Skin, hair
Associated channels	KI/BL	LR/GB	HT/SI/TB/PC	SP/ST	LU/LI

Abbreviations: BL, bladder; GB, gallbladder; HT, heart; KI, kidney; LI, large intestine; LR, liver; LU, lung; PC, pericardium; SI, small intestine; SP, spleen/pancreas; ST, stomach; TB, triple burner.

internal factor. Even today, red is still regarded as the color of fortune and happiness in China. Heat causes reddening and a burnt (bitter) taste. Summer is the associated season. Heat and joy affect especially the heart and the circulation. Correlated viscera are the triple burner and the small intestine. The sensory organ linked to the heart is the tongue. Joy must find expression, and when we are excited with joy, we tend to speak very quickly.

Well-known expressions that can serve as mnemonic aids are:
- "My heart is jumping for joy."
- "I am bursting with happiness."
- "When the heart is full, the tongue will speak."

Earth

Here, moistness, sweetness, aromatic smells, and the yellow color dominate. Sweetness refers to everything that is pleasing to the five sensory organs. Even the nipples, as the conduit to the fundamental source of food for infants, are located on the stomach channel. Late summer is the associated season. The spleen/pancreas and stomach are the correlated organs, in charge of food and the transformation of fluids, analogous to the function of the earth.

Well-known expressions that can serve as mnemonic aids are:
- "A fat belly, a lean brain."
- "I'm so worried my stomach is in knots."

The connection to the emotion "brooding/thinking" plays a role here. It is said that the spleen opens at the mouth and lips. Connective tissue and muscle mass are correlated with it.

Moisture causes sluggishness in processes of movement or thought, swelling, edemas, inertia, etc. Pain associated with this phase can be described as dull, unfocused, constant, numb, etc.

Metal

The defining energy here is dryness. Autumn is the associated season. Especially the respiratory tracts, lung, nose, and skin are affected by dryness. However, the viscus associated with this phase, the large intestine, is also not able to fulfill its function when exposed to excessive dryness. Constipation results.

A musty smell, a spicy-hot flavor that rises into the nose, and sadness and dissociation are associated with metal. Even today, white is the color of mourning in Asia. Dissociation and resistance are often typical reactions of a person in mourning.

Some expressions that can serve as mnemonic aids are:
- "A sigh of disappointment."
- "A chest heavy with sadness."

3.2.5 Relations between the Five Phases

The five phases cyclically produce water–wood–fire–earth–metal in sequential order, but they also have the function of controlling and promoting each other, thereby ensuring a harmonious equilibrium.

Sheng Cycle

The *sheng* cycle is the sequence of engendering, or the mother–child cycle. Within this cycle, each element produces its successor and promotes and supports it. Each phase thus gives nurturance (= mother) and at the same time receives nurturance (= child) (▶ Fig. 3.3).

Mother-water nurtures child-wood.
Mother-wood nurtures child-fire.
Mother-fire produces child-earth.
Mother-earth engenders child-metal.
Mother-metal gives birth to child-water.

Ke Cycle

The *ke* cycle, or restraining cycle, operates through the influence of each phase on the one after next. The grandmother not only controls the grandchild when the mother is no longer able to cope, but also regulates supportively if the child is weakened (▶ Fig. 3.3).

The notion of restraint should not be understood literally here because the organs and phases regulate each other by providing support, not by suppressing each other. In simpler terms, this means:

Water restrains/extinguishes fire.
Fire restrains/melts metal.
Metal restrains/splits wood.
Wood restrains/dams, penetrates earth.
Earth restrains/dams water.
The *ke* cycle guarantees that the equilibrium is maintained. An interdependent relationship results between the *sheng* and the *ke* cycles: under physiological conditions, this interrelation creates a continuously self-regulating equilibrium.

Cheng and *Wu* Cycles

These two cycles represent the disturbed equilibrium of the *sheng* and *ke* cycles (▶ Fig. 3.4):

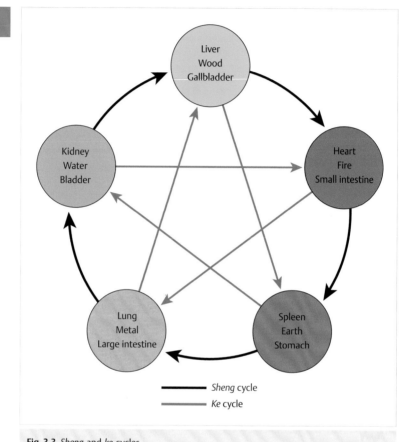

Fig. 3.3 *Sheng* and *ke* cycles.

***Cheng* Cycle** Cycle of overcoming, over-control, or invasion. It follows the same order as the restraint cycle. Here, one phase in fullness invasively controls the grandchild phase. The controlled phase is pathologically suppressed and weakened.

***Wu* Cycle** Insult (literal translation), mockery, or contempt sequence; rebellion.

It runs in the opposite direction to the restraint cycle: The phase to be restrained becomes pathologically stronger than the restraining phase and weakens it in a counterattack. Alternatively, the restraining phase is in a state of emptiness, in other words too weak, and is scorned in its restraint function and weakened by its grandchild phase.

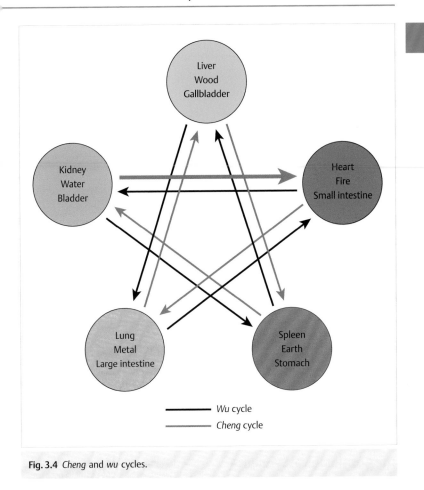

Fig. 3.4 *Cheng* and *wu* cycles.

Transfer Cycle

Invading climatic energy can lead to fullness in a control circuit and can then be passed on by means of induction according to the mother–child rule. In the supporting cycle, the energy runs especially toward the "opposite sex" between *yin* and *yang*.

In cases of emptiness, on the other hand, inhibition can increasingly withdraw energy from the mother through the mother–child cycle. Disorders that spread by the path of inhibition should always be regarded as more serious than those caused by induction.

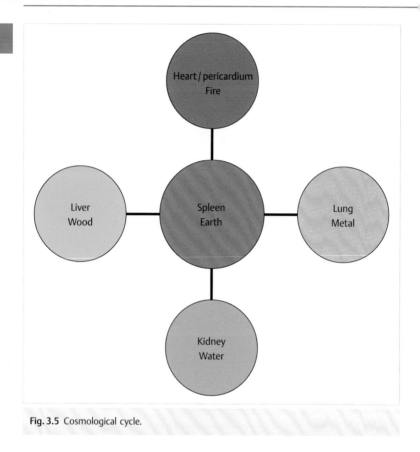

Fig. 3.5 Cosmological cycle.

The Cosmological Sequence

The cosmological sequence describes the five phases as stages in the cycle of the seasons (▶ Fig. 3.5).

This cycle is mentioned only rarely in the Western literature, in spite of its considerable clinical relevance:

- In the cosmological sequence, water forms the base for all other phases. Water is associated with the **kidney,** which, according to the theory of *zang fu* and the basic substances, constitutes the foundation of all

yang and *yin* in the body. The kidney governs water, which runs uphill to nourish the heart. The **heart** governs fire, which runs downhill to the kidney to warm it. This shows the fundamental interrelation between fire and water and reflects the equilibrium between *yin* and *yang*.

- The **spleen** and **stomach** occupy the central and neutral position in the middle of the cosmological sequence. Spleen and stomach provide the later heaven *qi* and thereby constitute the source of *qi* and blood.

- As the most important phase (by nurturing and transforming), **earth,** which is associated with the spleen and stomach, holds the central position. In this way, these organs also support the heart because they are its most important nurturers and supply it with *qi* and blood. Earth is not associated with any particular season but forms the neutral axis around which the seasons renew themselves. In Western books, earth is often correlated exclusively with late summer. In fact, though, it also corresponds to late winter, late autumn, and late spring.
- At the end of each season, the energy returns to earth, to regenerate itself.

4 The Channels

The channel system is comparable to a railroad, subway, or tramway network in a large city.

The flow of the network's electricity corresponds to the body's own *qi,* which is moving inside the organism along certain pathways, the so-called channels or *jing luo.*

The major channels are three-dimensional pathways that cover long routes close to the skin, like the transregional railroad systems on the periphery of cities, which traverse larger distances. The channels are often accompanied by blood vessels, nerves, and lymph vessels, just like the supply lines that support railway lines.

Different branches fork off from these superficial channel courses like tramways or subway lines that lead to destinations further inward and deeper in the city. These connect each channel to its associated organ, or the channels to each other or to certain body areas. Then there are further connecting lines, similar to bus lines with additional stops.

Acupuncture atlases only depict the superficial channels on which acupuncture points significant for diagnosis and therapy are located. The intermediate and underlying network remains "invisible," but supplies even the tiniest areas of the body with *qi* and blood. Here, the most obvious comparison would be with a taxi system, which is also not recorded on maps, but can, if necessary, provide transport to any point in the city.

The stops where the doors open to let passengers in or out, the acupuncture points, are specific places along the channels where resistance in the skin is measurably lower due to a higher number of nerve endings and capillaries. Tests have shown that this characteristic disappears after the death of the organism.

Looked at from the superficial layer directly underneath the skin regions, the following channels thus run at different depths from the outside to the inside:

- Closest to the surface are the cutaneous vessels.
- At the next depth are the tendinomuscular channels, the network vessels (*luo mai*), the main channels (*jing mai*), the extraordinary vessels (*qi jing ba mai: controlling vessel [ren mai], governing vessel [du mai], thoroughfare vessel [chong mai], girdling vessel [dai mai],* etc.), and the divergent channels (*bie luo*).
- At the lowest depth, we find the deep offshoots of the main channels and extraordinary vessels.

4.1 Function of the Channels

Keeping with the analogy of transport systems for passengers, materials, and energy in a large city, the function of the channels is to transport *qi* and blood through the entire body and to bind all bodily tissues together into a functioning community. They link inside and outside, right and left, above and below—similar to how transport systems link cities with each other. In the same way that cities establish communication with each other, so is a connection formed between practitioner and patient during acupuncture.

Additionally, the channels serve to protect the body against pathogenic factors that penetrate from outside. Here again we can draw a comparison to a road system on which emergency vehicles, police cars, and ambulances are able to move quickly, whenever necessary. This happens in each of the respective levels of the body traversed by the associated channel.

Among other functions, the network of channels serves as a barrier system against external pathogenic factors.

Another function of the channels is the reaction to "problems" that arise in the body, such as disorders of the channels themselves, the reflection of a viscus or bowel disorder in a channel, or the transmission of a process into another channel.

Yet another important role of the channels is to guide the *qi* into diseased areas to restore equilibrium there. The different properties of *qi* come into play as needed. The body's *qi* can perform a variety of tasks: It can transport, transform, contain/lift, protect, and nourish.

By stimulating acupuncture points, we can activate these processes and bring the required *qi* and blood to the areas of the body where they are needed.

4.2 Main Channels

The 12 main channels (***jing mai***) are the channels on which the most commonly used acupuncture points are located. They form the basis of this pocket atlas. Together with its associated organ, each channel forms a functional cycle, which then also determines its Western name.

 The six *yin* channels are linked to the viscera (*zang* or storage organs). The six *yang* channels are linked to the bowels (*fu* or hollow organs).

4.2.1 Course

The main channels run as pairs on both sides and symmetrically from cranial to caudal and from there back again along the body toward cranial. Each of the anterior and posterior extremities has three *yang* and three *yin* channels (▶ Table 4.1).

As a rule, we can say that the ***yin* channels** in general run along the **inside** of the extremities, while the ***yang* channels** are located on the **outside** of the legs and in the direction of the head. With the exception of the stomach channel (ST), they then all run along the back. Each of the 12 main channels has both this external course, on which the acupuncture points are located, as well as an internal course, which runs to the viscera and bowels in the body's cavity.

Table 4.1 *Yin* and *yang* channels on the foreleg and hind leg

	Foreleg		Hind leg	
	Main channels	Course	Main channels	Course
Yin channel	• Heart (HT) • Pericardium (PC) • Lung (LU)	Thorax foreleg (medial)	• Liver (LR) • Spleen/pancreas (SP) • Kidney (KI)	Hind leg (medial) → thorax or the flank
Yang channel	• Large intestine (LI) • Small intestine (SI) • Triple burner (TB)	Foreleg (craniolateral) → head	• Bladder (BL) • Gallbladder (GB) • Stomach (ST)	Eye → body → hind leg (lateral)

4.2.2 Nomenclature of the Main Channels

Unfortunately, the use of the same name for the channel and the associated anatomical organ, as is common in Western medicine, often leads to misunderstandings.

The reason for this is that, in Chinese medicine, the name of the organ does not refer to its anatomical structure but exclusively to its function. The term *"fei"* for "lung," for example, refers not to the two lobes of the lung that lie on the left and right side in the thorax, but to the entire respiratory function, which extends from the lung via the bronchial tubes to the nose and even over the skin. Western and Chinese organ names thus have little in common. Nevertheless, this atlas uses the shorter Western names.

In Chinese, the names of the channels consist of three parts:
1. Upper or lower extremity (hand/foot)
2. *Yin* or *yang* (in reference to the level)
3. Associated viscus or bowel

This results in the nomenclature listed in ▶ Table 4.2.

4.2.3 Relations between the Channels

Inside–Outside Relation

An inside–outside relation exists between the *yin* **channels** and *yang* **channels** that refers both to the anatomical location of the channels and to the associated paired viscera and bowels. The bladder channel, for example, runs along the posterior outside of the hind leg in the *yang* area, while the paired kidney channel is located on the posterior inside of the hind leg roughly across from it in the *yin* area.

The following channels thus stand in an inside–outside relation:
- **Forelegs**
  - Lung–large intestine
  - Pericardium–triple burner
  - Heart–small intestine

Table 4.2 Chinese and Western names of the 12 main channels

Chinese name	Western name (abbreviated)
Shou tai yin fei mai (hand *tai yin*)	Lung channel (LU)
Zu tai yin pi mai (foot *tai yin*)	Spleen/pancreas channel (SP)
Shou shao yin xin mai (hand *shao yin*)	Heart channel (HT)
Zu shao yin shen mai (foot *shao yin*)	Kidney channel (KI)
Shou jue yin xin bao mai (hand *jue yin*)	Pericardium channel (PC)
Zu jue yin gan mai (foot *jue yin*)	Liver channel (LR)
Shou tai yang xiao chang mai (hand *tai yang*)	Small intestine channel (SI)
Zu tai yang pang guang mai (foot *tai yang*)	Bladder channel (BL)
Shou shao yang san jiao mai (hand *shao yang*)	Triple burner channel (TB)
Zu shao yang dan mai (foot *shao yang*)	Gallbladder channel (GB)
Shou yang ming da chang mai (hand *yang ming*)	Large intestine channel (LI)
Zu yang ming wei mai (foot *yang ming*)	Stomach channel (ST)

- **Hind legs**
  - Kidney–bladder
  - Liver–gallbladder
  - Spleen/pancreas–stomach

Yang-Yang and *Yin-Yin* Relation

Each *yang* channel is paired with another *yang* channel, and each *yin* channel with another *yin* channel, from anterior to posterior in accordance with its anatomical location. The large intestine channel, for example, is thus linked to the stomach channel in *yang ming*. In this way, the 12 main channels form six pairs, which are usually referred to as **axes**. Each of these six pairs forms one of the "six layers," which carry a special significance in Chinese medicine.

The channels form the following axes:
- *Yin* axes
  - Lung–spleen/pancreas
  - Pericardium–liver
  - Heart–kidney
- *Yang* axes
  - Small intestine–bladder
  - Large intestine–stomach
  - Triple burner–gallbladder

Qi Cycles

The consecutive connections between the channels form the *qi* cycle through the main channels in the course of the day. The **flow of *qi*** begins with a *yin* channel at the thorax and runs into the paired *yang* channel at the foreleg.

From there, the *qi* flows to the face, where it passes over into the following *yang* channel, which runs to the back. At the foot, it then flows into the *yin* channel, which again brings the *qi* back forward to the thorax to start a new cycle. In this way, three

main cycles are formed, beginning with the lung, heart, and pericardium channels, respectively (▶ Fig. 4.1 and ▶ Fig. 4.2), which evenly supply the entire body.

The path of *qi* through the body along the main channels follows three major cycles:
- First cycle: LU-LI-ST-SP
- Second cycle: HT-SI-BL-KI
- Third cycle: PC-TB-GB-LR

4.2.4 The Organ Clock

Within the three cycles and from one cycle to the next, *qi* is passed on consecutively through the 24 hours of the day. Each channel contains the maximum *qi* for 2 hours before the state of maximum energy is transmitted to the following channel (▶ Fig. 4.3). As a result, each channel also has a certain time during which it contains only a minimum amount of energy.

 During the peak times of each functional cycle, specific related disturbances or pathogenic influences manifest most distinctly.

4.3 Divergent Channels

The divergent channels are offshoots of the 12 main channels without their own points. They branch off from their main channel at specific locations and follow their own course from there on:

The **yang divergent channels** of the *yang* channels:
- Depart from the main channels at the extremities
- Enter the connected viscus or bowel and then the paired *yin* or *yang* viscus or bowel
- Come back to the surface at the throat or face, to reconnect with the main channel

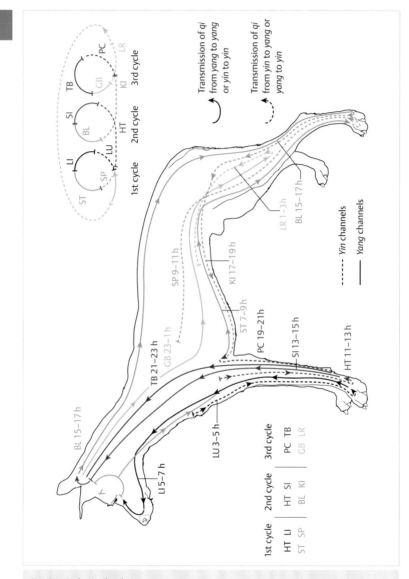

Fig. 4.1 Cycles in the dog.

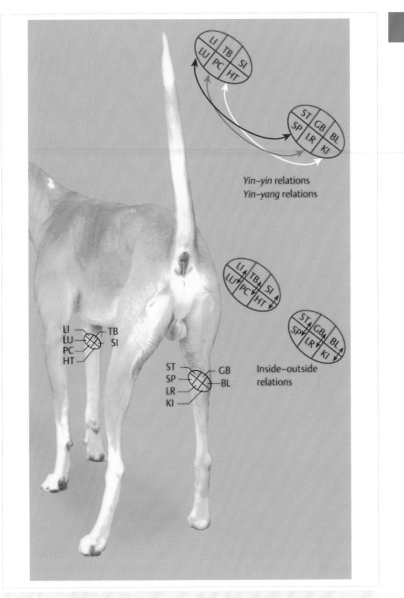

Fig. 4.2 *Yin* and *yang* correlations of the channels according to their location.

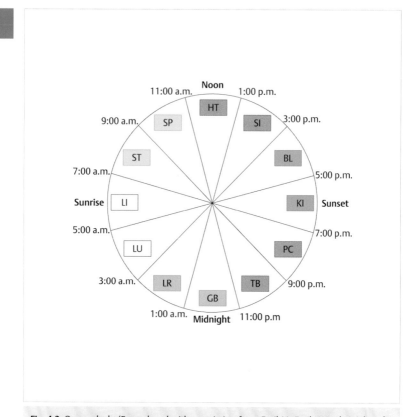

Fig. 4.3 Organ clock. (Reproduced with permission from Ergil M, Ergil K. Pocket Atlas of Chinese Medicine. Stuttgart-New York: Thieme Publishers; 2009.)

The **yin divergent channels** of the yin channels:

- Depart from the main channels at the extremities;
- Partly enter the associated viscus;
- Run together with the paired yang divergent channels;
- Then connect to the paired yang main channel itself.

The pathways of the divergent channels and their connections between the main channels and the organs or certain body regions explain the effect of several acupuncture points located on the main channels, which otherwise would not have any connection there.

The divergent channels perform several functions:

- They provide for the stable connection between paired yin and yang channels and between the viscera and bowels.
- They transport qi and blood to the head and face.

- They supply body regions that are not supplied by the main channels.
- They link main channels to body regions that they do not reach directly.

4.4 Extraordinary Vessels

The eight extraordinary vessels (*qi jing ba mai*; ▶ Table 4.3) function as reservoirs and compensatory vessels for *qi* and blood and follow their own course. They intersect with the main channels, also connecting these to each other; however, they lie deeper within the body. The extraordinary vessels protect the body.

Each of the extraordinary vessels has an acupuncture point on the main channel that serves as its **"opener"** or **"activator,"** and a point that functions as **"closer"** or **"coupler"** when it is needled contralaterally after the opener (▶ Table 4.4). This form of acupuncture activates the respective extraordinary vessel and its highly specific characteristics.

Table 4.3 The eight extraordinary vessels and their functions

Extraordinary vessel	Function
Governing vessel (*du mai*)*	Regulates *qi* in all *yang* channels because it connects them to each other at GV-14
Yang qiao mai (*yang* springing vessel)	Links the bladder, gallbladder, stomach, large intestine, and small intestine channels and thereby controls the activity of the body
Controlling vessel (*ren mai*, "sea of *yin*")*	Links all *yin* channels, and as the "sea of *yin*" regulates all *yin* channels
Yin qiao mai (*yin* springing vessel)	Links the kidney and bladder channels and controls emotional balance
Thoroughfare vessel (*chong mai*, "sea of blood and of the 12 main channels")*	Links the stomach and kidney channels and also strengthens the connection between the controlling and governing vessels, which both originate in the pelvic area and run dorsally and ventrally to the front
Yin wei mai (*yin* linking vessel)	Influences the inside of the entire body by linking the kidney, spleen, and liver channels as well as the controlling vessel
Girdling vessel (*dai mai*)	Links all 12 main channels, governing and controlling vessels like a broad belt in the hip area
Yang wei mai (*yang* linking vessel)	Influences the outside of the entire body by linking the bladder, gallbladder, triple burner, stomach, and small intestine channels as well as the governing vessel

* The thoroughfare vessel (*chong mai*), controlling vessel (*ren mai*), and governing vessel (*du mai*) circulate defense *qi* (*wei qi*) through the thorax, abdomen, and back and thus create a defense mechanism against external pathogenic influences.

Table 4.4 Opener and coupler of the eight extraordinary vessels

	Opener	Coupler
Governing vessel (*du mai*)	SI-3	BL-62
Yang qiao mai (*yang* springing vessel)	BL-62	SI-3
Controlling vessel (*ren mai*)	LU-7	KI-6
Yin qiao mai (*yin* springing vessel)	KI-6	LU-7
Thoroughfare vessel (*chong mai*)	SP-4	PC-6
Yin wei mai (*yin* linking vessel)	PC-6	SP-4
Girdling vessel (*dai mai*)	GB-41	TB-5
Yang wei mai (*yang* linking vessel)	TB-5	GB-41

4.5 Network Vessels (*Luo Mai*)

Each of the 12 main channels has a *luo* point where the associated *luo* or network vessel originates. From there it runs with one branch as the **transverse luo vessel** to the paired *yin* or *yang* channel. The other branch continues as the **longitudinal luo vessel** relatively on the surface. From there on, these vessels have their own course.

The *luo* vessels strengthen the inside–outside connection of paired channels as well as the connection to the viscera and bowels.

There are 15 network vessels: 12 to the main channels and then one each to the controlling vessel (*ren mai*) and the governing vessel (*du mai*), as well as the large network vessel of the spleen, which branches off at SP-21 (▶ Table 4.5).

4.6 Tendinomuscular Channels

The tendinomuscular channels run superficially on the periphery along the lines of the major muscles and muscle groups, including the tendons and ligaments. They remain peripheral and do not penetrate to the viscera and bowels in the interior of the body. They are named after the main channels that they are linked to and always originate in the extremities. From there, they run toward the trunk and head, approximately following the course of the main channel while being broader than the main channel.

The tendinomuscular channels either manifest disturbances of the main channel or are themselves disturbed by external pathogenic influences (e.g., injuries). There are no specific points associated with them. They are most effectively treated by stimulating the *ah shi* points (corresponding roughly to the trigger or pain points; see *Ah Shi Points*), cupping, massage, etc.

4.7 Cutaneous Vessels

To supply each of the distally located body regions with *qi* and blood, the organism has at its disposal numerous tiny branches of the major vessels. These offshoots are known as cutaneous vessels. They do not have their own points but are reached by needling the points on the main channels to which they are linked.

Table 4.5 Course of the network vessels

Main channel	Course	
	From	To
Lung channel	LU-7	Palmar surface and thorax
Large intestine channel	LI-6	Jaws, teeth, ear
Stomach channel	ST-40	Throat, neck, head
Spleen/pancreas channel	SP-4	Abdomen, stomach, intestines
Heart channel	HT-5	Heart, dorsum of the tongue, eye
Small intestine channel	SI-7	Shoulder
Bladder channel	BL-58	Kidney channel
Kidney channel	KI-4	Along the kidney channel to the perineum and lumbar vertebrae
Pericardium channel	PC-6	Pericardium and heart
Triple burner channel	TB-5	Meeting point with the pericardium channel in the thorax
Gallbladder channel	GB-37	Back of the foot
Liver channel	LV-5	Genitals, running across abdomen
Controlling vessel	CV-15	Running across abdomen
Governing vessel	GV-1	Along the lateral spinal column up to the roof of the skull. Shoulder blades, joining the bladder channel and penetrating into the spinal column
Spleen network channel	SP-21	Through thorax and lateral rib area

4.8 Cutaneous Regions

The cutaneous regions lie on top of the channels in the skin, are linked to them, and can indicate more deeply lying disturbances; for example, by discoloration of the skin.

5 Psychoemotional Foundations of Veterinary Acupuncture

5.1 Animal Psychology in Traditional Chinese Veterinary Medicine (TCVM)

The inseparability of physical and psychological problems is a foundational principle of Chinese medicine. In this context, *shen*, *qi*, and *jing* are the "three treasures" that embody heaven, earth, and the living beings in between (▶ Table 5.1).

There is a quote by Li Dongyuan that can be roughly translated in this way: "*Qi* is the ancestor of *shen*, and *jing* is the child of *qi*. As such, *qi* is the root of both *jing* and *shen*. How great is this *qi*! When it collects, it produces *jing*. When *jing* collects, it keeps the *shen* healthy." The absolute potential of *shen* materializes by means of *jing*, and in the context of this tension *qi* manifests all living being on earth. Life thus means the transformation from fire to water. The *Dao* is understood as the path or plan of life. It comes from the *shen* and can only be realized and achieved when the *qi* flows smoothly in one's life because the five elements (or five phases) are able to operate in balance. The polarity between *yin* and *yang* is what makes the creation of *qi* possible in the first place. It is only through tension that electricity can flow, that energy can work.

The five elements metal, water, wood, fire, and earth form the basic elements of the universe and the world. They generate each other and influence and regulate each other. The five phases of change form a dynamic cycle, in which one phase continuously changes over into the next one. At first sight, this monad appears to represent merely the relationship between two forces, at second sight, a fourfold system. This system forms the foundation for the system of the five phases of change. Depending on the nature of each element, its *yin* and *yang* aspects shift, which induces change in the associated *qi* as the effective vector. The condition of individual elements also changes the composition of the *qi*. These shifts can change the flow of *qi*, its direction, its force, and hence the balance. The five storage organs (*zang* or *yin* organs) produce the associated energy of their emotions and are connected to them, but can also be disturbed by them. Every excess or deficiency, also in relation to the emotions, damages the associated organ system or disturbs the circulation of *qi* and blood. Emotions are referred to as internal pathogenic factors (see Internal Pathogenic Factors (p. 38)).

They have the greatest influence on the flow of *qi* and therefore on the health of

Table 5.1 The three treasures

"Three treasures"	Meaning	Relation	Quality
Shen	Fire—spirit, potential	Heaven	Highest *yang* energy
Qi	Living beings—thinking, actualization	Earth	Five elements (or five phases)
Jing	Inheritance—kidney, DNA, matter	Water	Greatest *yin* energy

the body. In this context, shock, fear, and deep apprehensiveness are such strongly blocking energies that they can disturb every other emotion and every organ. When emotions are not balanced or released, this leads to stagnation, and that can lead to illness.

 The secret to balanced emotions is transformation.

When all emotions are balanced, the flow of *qi* is most abundant, and the tension between the poles is reduced. We become closer to the *Dao*, the balance of the poles fire and water. Matter and spirit become one. But what is a feeling to begin with? The character for emotion is *qing* and contains the characters for heart, life, and juicy grass. This rapidly changeable, sensitive force can thus always exert an influence on one of the five aspects of the *shen* in the heart: thought, consciousness, insight, memory, and sleep. To achieve a sense of oneness, the heart has to be completely empty of disturbing emotions. The word "emotion" contains the notion of movement. Movement is produced through tension, and this flow corresponds to the *qi*. Because emotions are formed in the *zang fu*, we can visualize each organ as a steel drum. Each one tuned differently with a different sound pattern that can be struck. In response, these patterns resonate, and the resulting frequencies produce different sounds. These sounds in turn are the emotions that are supposed to regulate the *qi* flow. The *qi* flows along the channels, and the emotion that it embodies is perceived as a feeling in the associated *zang fu* or sense organ because of the phenomenon of frequency resonance. The emotions then operate like filters that determine how the external reality is perceived internally by

the sense organs. All emotions move the spirit and the thoughts in their own way, and every emotion is responsible for different activities. This makes it obvious once again how an acupuncturist can never separate the treatment of the body from that of the psyche.

5.2 The Effects of Points at the Psychological Level

Acupuncture moves earthbound *qi* in the conduits and thus has an obvious connection to the material body. But most points also have a connection to psychological energies and therefore also work at a different level. Point names give clear hints. Thus, they also operate in the energy field of the body, which surrounds it. In animals, this emotional level of energy is particularly strong (▶ Fig. 5.1). Traditional Chinese Medicine (TCM) recognizes different levels of consciousness and aspects of the soul in humans. The inseparability of physical and psychological problems becomes clear in the correlation of *hun*, *po*, *shen*, *jing*, and *qi* with the organs. But we can also use the theory of the five elements to describe types that can be associated with clearly defined psychological properties. The discussion on whether animals have a consciousness and what it is that ultimately distinguishes humans decisively from animals is an inexhaustible topic.

Consciousness is the knowledge of differentiation and of the extent of one's own self in relation to the environment and to other living beings.

In order to distinguish animal consciousness from human consciousness, we can follow Hediger and subdivide between primary and secondary consciousness.

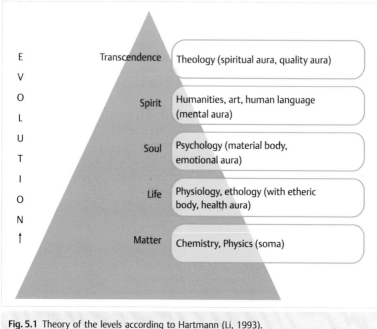

E
V
O
L
U
T
I
O
N
↑

Transcendence — Theology (spiritual aura, quality aura)

Spirit — Humanities, art, human language (mental aura)

Soul — Psychology (material body, emotional aura)

Life — Physiology, ethology (with etheric body, health aura)

Matter — Chemistry, Physics (soma)

Fig. 5.1 Theory of the levels according to Hartmann (Li, 1993).

Secondary consciousness is the ability to realize awareness, i.e., to reflect on it (also reflexive awareness).

The German philosopher Nicolai Hartmann (1882–1950) divided the energetic levels of humans and animals chronologically in accordance with evolution. As such, animals in general possess the first three levels, while the subsequent spiritual level is said to be limited to humans alone. Science, art, and human language are found in this realm. Heini Hediger adds an additional fifth level of transcendence above that. At this level, we deal with life after death, abstract and philosophical foundations, as well as theology.

Apparently, it is thus possible that we interact and communicate with animals on three of the five levels. A necessary prerequisite, which also applies for a successful acupuncture treatment, is that we resonate at the relevant energetic level. To do this, sensitivity and empathic feeling and acting are necessary.

5.3 Five Element Types in Dogs and Cats According to Their Emotional Behavior

The evaluation of healthy behavior is informed by the animal species, age, living conditions, and "use" of an animal. Type associations in accordance with the five elements is one tool used by Chinese medicine, in order to better evaluate and understand the patients, and to classify their behavior more clearly as physiological or pathological. This concerns hereditary predispositions and sensitivities.

5.3.1 Water

Emotional Water types tend toward caution and attentiveness toward potential danger. General fears, fear of the unknown, extreme worrying and tension, fear of injury and pain, sensitivity to noise and being gun-shy, as well as black depression can visit them. The energy is directed inward. Self-preservation and the will to survive are connected to the functional system of water. (When the world collapses, follow a water type, because they will always come out the other end and survive!) When there is a reason for fear, water types flee and run off into the distance. When water types become unsettled, they freeze into a proverbial "pillar of salt." On the other hand, though, water types have a strong will and enormous perseverance when they have set their mind on something. The pursuit of a distinct goal gives them security. In a fight, the functional systems *shen* and *gan* join forces to attack (fear biter). When a fear-based paralysis occurs in an attack, this is connected to a weakness in *dan*. When panic results, it is connected to a weakness in *xin*. The ability to detect the smallest changes in the emotional environment is the strength of the kidney.

Proper Handling When you want to win over a water type, you absolutely have to give them security for the right path. Literally take such animals by the hand, lead them bravely, and treat them with great care. Never give water types a feeling of

insecurity. This can lead to unpredictable panic reactions. The unknown has to be approached slowly, and you always have to be prepared for fear reactions to suddenly occurring noises. But there is also strength to be found here in their adaptability and a great capacity for learning and understanding.

5.3.2 Wood

Emotional Wood types tend toward dominant behavior and independent decisions. Imagination and intensity are their strength. Their energy is directed upward. But changes in the daily routine are not appreciated. Instead, they bring initiative and inspiration to their work. Wood types require exercise for their muscles. Pauses in exercise cause their energy to pile up and can lead to unpredictable releases. When they feel confined and constricted in their ability to move, they can respond with claustrophobia. But at a minimum, they react with signs of stress and being upset.

Subsequent attacks are not infrequent. Quick comprehension, accuracy, and speed in both physical as well as intellectual and emotional abilities depend on the condition of the liver. The most common emotional disturbance with physical effects is connected to the liver system. Liver function suffers quickly as the result of persistent rage, irascibility, fury, depression, frustration, or anger, and is a sign of an imbalance in wood, or in the functional system of the gallbladder. In charge of initiative, innovation, forward movement, and planned action under healthy circumstances, wood energy leads to new challenges. Finishing up tasks, however, is not its strength.

Proper Handling Ambition makes wood types enthusiastic athletes, combining a need for exercise with a desire to win. For this goal, they sometimes ignore injuries. A regular routine of daily life and training with consistent exercise works best for wood types. They thrive best in both physical and emotional terms when they have completed their set "task" and in this way fulfilled their "plan." They do not have a need for cuddling and prefer a stronger touch. As reward for concentrated work, they benefit from free movement.

5.3.3 Fire

Emotional Fire types need friends, otherwise they quickly feel lonely. When in doubt, they will do everything for their best friend. Their energy is directed to the outside. They want to be the center of your world, and when they feel neglected, they will demand your attention emphatically. This can have the effect that fire types open themselves up uncritically to any contact, which then leads to the risk of disappointment. It is possible that the animal no longer permits outside contacts due to relationship problems and disappointments. Vitality, zest for life, happiness, excitements, cheerfulness, and pleasure are positive fire traits, that can flip into hysteria, despair, excessive excitement, and fear of not being loved, or fear of sexuality, when they become unbalanced. Pronounced sentimentality is a human sign of fire quality. Fire types are animals that call out loudly when they notice their caregiver, as well as those who love communication with their fellow species.

Proper Handling You can always make fire types happy with toys. This playful behavior can be put to good use as motivation for training. In training, it is essential to take pleasure and playfulness into consideration. Fire types are happy to "work" with you when it brings joy to them and to you and feels like fun. They can get excited about things and practically be burning to

do something. The best rewards are play sessions, loud joy, and clearly expressed enthusiasm. Never dwell on a problem for a long time. This quickly makes fire types bored, so that they can then promptly get upset about the most trivial thing to compensate for it and overreact dangerously when they can find even the smallest excuse. Quickly changing tasks with variable training units are the best guarantee for keeping such an animal under control and, most importantly, motivated.

5.3.4 Earth

Emotional Earth types are tied to reality, are centered, like company, and enjoy taking care of small or young animals or of groups. They welcome groups of children as much as the new young animal in a pack. Earth types carefully look after their offspring and, when thrown off balance, can become overprotective and not give their offspring enough freedom. Their other strengths are reliability, security, and stability. They have an eye for the needs of others, but can become unbalanced when they lose their self-confidence. Then they sink into brooding, worrying, or self-doubt. Earth types try to give everything that is asked of them. Fear of failure, overwork, and the absence of a secure place in the group damage the spleen *qi*, which can have physical results.

Proper Handling Food is the best motivation for earth types. A mini break with a snack from your pocket is the most certain sign for earth types that they have solved the last task to your full satisfaction. And in general, it is most important for earth types that they please the human and perform everything as correctly as possible. They are not so quick in their thinking and reactions, and it is therefore good to give them one task to solve after another and not to challenge them too much. In that case, they worry too much and fret that they were unable to satisfy you. Fear of failure is the greatest problem for imbalances in earth. This blocks them and makes everything more difficult. This can become a problem in terms of success in learning and in test situations, but also with partners and breeding. It is not infrequent that this leads to obsessive-compulsive neuroses, as the result of the tendency of earth personalities to get stuck in permanent brooding with no way out, in conjunction with the need to do everything correctly. Another aspect is their unconditional motivation. Aggression and stress are wood properties that can cause problems for earth types and thereby impair the function of the stomach and spleen-pancreas.

5.3.5 Metal

Emotional Metal types have a tendency to put up boundaries. Their energies are directed downward. They like to make their own decisions but do not want to take the lead. They prefer to stand on their own and watch others from a certain distance. They are stable personalities, and it is a good choice to regard them as special. They are conscious of their outer appearance and tend to always look clean and neat. If you fail to recognize their unique value, you will not be able to connect with them at all. They will literally shake you off like water on the outside. This is intensified even further when they experience grief. They do not process losses well. The dramatic loss of an offspring, the death of a fellow member of their species, or separation from their beloved caregiver can trigger grief that can build up over many years. This can even have the effect that metal types angrily reject any kind of attempted rapprochement. Emotional imbalances like grief, worry, loneliness, or a feeling of abandonment damage the

strength of the lung and empty its *qi*. If deficiency in metal prevents the control of wood, aggressive tendencies can get even worse. Fear of being alone is a huge issue! Breathing in and breathing out, giving and taking, accepting and letting go—these are *the* concerns of metal, of the lung, and the large intestine.

Proper Handling Metal types do great with training and expect absolutely precise instructions. When these do not come, they act as if you were speaking Chinese and, when in doubt, do not do anything, and with an almost arrogant attitude. They train their human partner to work with precision, and when the human recognizes their specialness, as they themselves perceive it, they will do anything for them.

Thus spoke the fatalist:
You must become what you are.
Resistance is futile.
The master of all life
Granted you your wish and willfulness
Already at the Beginning
Here a yes, and there a no
To be exactly thus.
(Wilhelm Busch)

5.4 The Role of Pathogenic Factors

Chinese medicine not only offers the possibility to get to know your animal better and thereby also to improve your ability to work with them, but also a chance to recognize imbalances as such and to treat them. Qualified acupuncturists with sufficient experience can often restore the basic energetic balance with just a few treatments. Physical and emotional problems can be successfully treated with this modality. In real life, all humans and animals always exhibit at least two or even three different characteristic qualities. But in most cases, one happens to be dominant and clearly recognizable, when we look closely.

Among all pathogenic factors, the internal factors, or in other words, the emotional factors, are precisely those that have the greatest influence on the formation of illness. In accordance with their nature, excessive joy, anger, brooding, worry, fear, fright, and grief can block the *qi* in each of the channel systems.

Emotional disharmony leads to disturbed behavior in the environment, which leads to disharmony in relationships, which in turn gives rise to disturbed emotions. In this context, *zang fu* disharmony can function both as a trigger for emotional imbalances and as their result (▶ Fig. 5.2).

"Emotional imbalance influences the harmonic function of the *zang fu*, the formation of substances and their transport into all regions of the body" (J. Ross).

In addition to influences during the life of an individual, the emotional stability of the patient can also be affected by problems or negative energies that happened during the time in the womb.

According to chapter 8 of the *Suwen*, anger, indignation, fear, worry, grief, and fright (The Seven Emotions) can damage the source *qi* in such a way that the entire *zang fu* system is negatively affected. If these seven "passions" or stagnation in the heart produce racing rage or excessive *yin* fire, the *shen* no longer receives nourishment from the heart, the channels contain nothing but fire, and the seven spirits leave their form.

But a *shen* disturbance can also result from inadequate processing of food due to *wei* or *pi* imbalances. This means that we only have to harmonize the spleen and stomach in order to soothe and relax the source *qi* in the stomach. This benefits all *zang fu*, since there is once again a sufficient supply of *yuan qi* for all of them.

The consistent functioning of the *zang fu* is necessary not only for all the physical processes but also because it is responsible for the function of the nine openings and thereby for the psychological state of the patient.

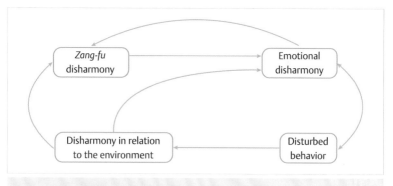

Fig. 5.2 Vicious cycle of emotional disharmony (Ross, 1986).

In TCM, *gan* and *xin* are the two *zang* organs that have the greatest effect on the harmonic interplay of the emotions. They are responsible for an adequate and calm reaction to stimuli from the environment.

"When the heart is free from rigidity and stagnation because of joy, beautiful presents, nice weather, healing life circumstances, delicious food, or a beautiful sight, the patient will be happy and recover from the illness" (Li).

Suggested Readings

Claude Larre JS. Survey of Traditional Chinese Medicine. Paris: Institut Ricci; 1986

Eul-Matern C. Akupunktur bei Pferdekrankheiten. Stuttgart: Sonntag; 2013

Eul-Matern C. Akupunktur bei Krankheiten von Hund und Katze. Stuttgart: Sonntag; 2015

Hediger H. Tier verstehen. Erkenntnisse eines Tierpsychologen. München: Kindler; 1984

Li D-Y. The Treatise on the Spleen and Stomach: A Translation of the Pi Wei Lun. Blue Poppy Press; 1993

Müller JV. Den Geist Verwurzeln. München: Müller und Steinicke; 2004

Ross J. Zang Fu: The Organ Systems of Traditional Chinese Medicine. Churchill Livingstone; 1986

6 Traditional Chinese Veterinary Medicine Diagnostics

Traditional Chinese diagnostics (*bianzheng*) consists of:
- *bian* = differentiate and identify;
- *zheng* = describe the type or pattern of the disorder.

> ❗ In Traditional Chinese Veterinary Medicine (TCVM), we observe all the clinical signs and enlist them to determine the diagnosis. Thereby, we also include signs that (from the Western perspective) appear not to belong to the actual pathological process.

We attempt to create a connection between:
- Existing symptoms;
- One or more functional cycles;
- The different aspects of *yin* and *yang*; and
- Environmental influences.

Given the increasing alienation of our daily lives from a natural environment, it seems more important than ever today to include the influence of the environment in diagnosis and treatment. Anything that alienates the organism from nature has the ability to disrupt the equilibrium of its natural energy system.

The seasonal or climatic conditions under which a disorder initially arose are as important for diagnosis as the living conditions or the particular development of the disease. Also significant are the time of day and/or season during which a problem manifests with particular clarity.

Like Chinese human medicine, Chinese veterinary medicine has also continually developed over several thousand years. Today, the differences between their methods are negligible.

The **nine most important theories** (▶ Table 6.1) by which we can make a TCVM diagnosis are as follows:
1. Pathogenic factors (see Pathogenic Factors Diagnosis [p. 36])
2. The eight guiding principles (see Eight Principles Diagnosis [p. 38])
3. The viscera and bowels (see Organ Diagnosis [p. 39])
4. The six levels (see Six Levels Diagnosis [*Shang Han Lun*] [p. 39])
5. The four aspects *wei*, *qi*, *ying*, and *xue* (see Four Aspects Diagnosis [*Wen Bing*] [p. 39])
6. The triple burner (see Triple Burner Diagnosis [*San Jiao Bian Zheng*] [p. 40])
7. The channels (see Channel Diagnosis [p. 40])
8. The five basic substances (see Five Basic Substances Diagnosis [p. 40])
9. The five phases (see Five Phases Diagnosis [p. 41])

No symptom or pathological sign is considered in isolation. The interrelations between individual symptoms are eminently important for the diagnosis.

The choice of applicable treatment principle depends in each case on the applied diagnostic system. This means that it is impossible, for example, to treat liver *qi* stagnation (= organ pathology) by removing internal wind (= pathogenic factor). Instead, it is important here to move *qi* in the area of the functional cycle liver, to resolve the stagnation.

6.1 Pathogenic Factors Diagnosis

This theory describes the ways in which supplemental factors such as internal or external

Table 6.1 Survey of the nine diagnostic systems of TCVM

Diagnostic system	Brief description	Applicability
Pathogenic factors	• External pathogenic factors: 　– Wind 　– Cold 　– Heat 　– Summer heat 　– Dampness 　– Dryness • Internal pathogenic factors: 　– Emotions • Other pathogenic factors: 　– Hunger 　– Overexertion	• Any acute disorder • Often present in excess syndromes
Eight guiding principles = basis of Chinese diagnosis	• Basis of pattern differentiation • Four pairs—six basic patterns 　– Yin–yang 　– Inside–outside 　– Repletion–vacuity 　– Cold–heat	• Basis of TCVM diagnosis • Any disorder
Organ patterns = the "heart" of Chinese diagnostics	• Each viscus or bowel has its own excess–deficiency/heat–cold pattern	• Chronic (internal) disorders • Generalized weakness • Geriatrics
Six levels	• *Tai yang–tai yin* • *Yang ming–shao yin* • *Shao yang–jue yin*	• Chronic inflammatory disorders • Cold-induced disorders • External disorders
Four aspects	• *Wei* • *Qi* • *Ying* • *Xue*	• Infectious diseases • Any disorder that begins with fever and progresses toward the inside if not stopped • External disorders
Triple burner patterns	• Upper burner • Middle burner • Lower burner	• External disorders • Beginning with fever and progressing from the upper to the lower burner
Channel patterns	• Twelve main channels • Eight extraordinary vessels	• Musculoskeletal problems
Qi, blood, and *jin ye*	• Pathogenic changes in qi, blood, and bodily fluids	• Chronic internal disorders • Endocrine imbalances
Five phases	• Water • Wood • Fire • Earth • Metal	• Any disorder

influences can disturb the equilibrium in the body. At this point, the practitioner realizes with particular poignancy the need for advice on dietetics and rearing conditions.

We distinguish between external, internal, and other pathogenic factors.

6.1.1 External Pathogenic Factors

We can distinguish between six climatic factors that can cause symptoms and signs of disease in accordance with their specific properties:
1. Wind
2. Cold
3. Heat
4. Summer heat
5. Dampness
6. Dryness

External pathogenic factors can be used to describe not only weather-related influences, but also bacterial, viral, or parasitic changes.

The symptoms caused by pathogenic factors are a manifestation of the conflict between the organism's *wei qi* and the pathogenic factor, and reveal the picture that results from this fight. As such, what determines the picture of the illness is not just the nature of the invader.

6.1.2 Internal Pathogenic Factors

(See also *Chapter 5 Psychoemotional Foundations of Veterinary Acupuncture*).

These are related to the influence of psychoemotional strain on the organism:
• Rage/irritation: wood
• Joy/hectic: fire
• Fear/fright: water
• Brooding/worrying: earth
• Sadness/grief: metal

The name of the pattern is based on the affected phase and organ (e.g., deficiency in metal due to grief).

6.1.3 Other Pathogenic Factors

The other pathogenic factors are neither unequivocally external nor unequivocally internal. These, for example, include psychological or physical overexertion, the wrong diet, or too many litters.

6.2 Eight Principles Diagnosis

The method of identifying patterns in accordance with the eight guiding principles is known as *ba gang*. The eight guiding principles characterize and elucidate in detail the possible manifestations of *yin* and *yang*:
1. Basic principles: *yin–yang*
2. Localization: inside–outside
3. Quality: cold–heat
4. Quantity: deficiency–excess

These differentiations provide the eight guiding principles. By assigning the signs detected, the practitioner creates a differentiated Chinese diagnosis. One example for such a diagnosis would be internal cold/excess.

Pattern identification in accordance with the eight principles is the basis for all other diagnostic options.

 Physiology, pathology, diagnosis, and therapy in TCVM all ultimately deal with the relationship between *yin* and *yang* and disturbances thereof.

6.3 Organ Diagnosis

Patterns of the viscera and bowels are based on the symptoms and disease signs that arise when *qi* and blood in the internal organs are thrown off-balance. This method is applied mostly for internal and chronic conditions, but also includes external and acute patterns.

In clinical practice, many symptoms do not always manifest at the same time. The art of diagnosis lies in our ability to recognize the existing disharmony on the basis of a few disease signs. The organ patterns should not be understood as diseases in the Western sense but as manifestations of a prevailing energetic and substantial disharmony. They have no connection to Western organ syndromes.

In clinical practice, several patterns can appear simultaneously in a single case. Several viscera or bowels can be affected, for example, or one organ can have different patterns. An example of this would be the simultaneous occurrence of liver *qi* stagnation and spleen *qi* deficiency.

6.4 Six Levels Diagnosis (*Shang Han Lun*)

The six levels model is one of the oldest diagnostic methods. It describes disorders that are caused by **cold.** Carried by wind, cold invades the body. In most of these cases, we are dealing with external conditions. Depending on the severity of the cold, the patient's state of resistance, and the chronological progression of the disorder, the cold leads to a clearly defined disease picture.

The cold can penetrate further into the body along the following six channel levels (see *Yang–Yang* and *Yin–Yin* Relation (p.21)), developing typical disease signs:

- *Yang* levels
    - Small intestine–bladder = *tai yang*
    - Triple burner–gallbladder = *shao yang*
    - Large intestine–stomach = *yang ming*
- *Yin* levels
    - Lung–spleen/pancreas = *tai yin*
    - Heart–kidney = *shao yin*
    - Pericardium–liver = *jue yin*

The first three (*yang*) levels indicate patterns in which the body is strongly resisting the pathogenic factor. The three *yin* levels represent patterns in which the *zheng qi* is already weakened.

Patterns of *shang han* conditions develop relatively slowly over the course of one or several days.

The development of six-level patterns can occur in three ways:

1. Regular development from the outside to the inside: *Tai yang-shao yang-yang ming-tai yin-shao yin-jue yin.*
2. Skipping levels: Under certain unfavorable conditions, one or more levels can be skipped and the pathogenic factor can move deeper into the body (e.g., from *tai yang* to *yang ming* or even *tai yin*).
3. Direct attack: When the body's resistance is weak, the pathogen can arrive directly in the *yin* layers on the inside.

6.5 Four Aspects Diagnosis (*Wen Bing*)

Wei-qi-ying-xue patterns (four-aspect patterns) are highly acute febrile diseases that are caused by external **heat factors.** By describing them precisely, we are able to distinguish and treat arising febrile diseases. They proceed acutely and damage *yin*, fluids, and blood.

Depending on the season, we observe different pathogens and syndromes. The pathogen can, for example, pass through the mouth and nose or skin and muscles into the organism and initially affect the exterior level of *wei qi*. The disease begins with a sudden onset and proceeds rapidly with heat symptoms.

Table 6.2 Diseases according to the four-aspects pattern

Stage	Level	Location
1	*Wei*	Superficial, muscles, joints
2	*Qi*	Lung, stomach, large intestine
3	*Ying*	Central nervous system, heart, *shen*, pericardium
4	*Xue*	Hemorrhage

Depending on the strength of the pathogenic factor and the organism's defense *qi*, it penetrates deeply into the body and damages first the *jin ye* and then the blood. It can then affect the levels of *qi*, *ying*, and *xue* in sequence (▶ Table 6.2). Recovery would proceed in the opposite order.

6.6 Triple Burner Diagnosis (*San Jiao Bian Zheng*)

The basis for classifying patterns according to the triple burner (*san jiao*) is the three-part division of the body:
1. Upper burner: heart, lung
2. Middle burner: stomach, spleen, liver
3. Lower burner: kidney, bladder, small intestine, large intestine

Triple burner patterns arise due to exogenous pathogenic factors. In general, we distinguish between cold-induced and heat-induced conditions. A comparison with the six levels model (see Six Levels Diagnosis (p. 39)) is suitable here. Under conditions of the six levels model, the movement runs from below (*tai yang*, bladder channel,

water) to above. In triple burner patterns, the pathogen enters from above via the mouth and nose. The symptoms run from above to below, according to set patterns.

6.7 Channel Diagnosis

Channel pathologies are exclusively concerned with externally discernible problems of the 12 main channels and eight extraordinary vessels. Because channels and organs form an energy-based unit but certainly also function separately, disharmonies in the channels can affect the organs and vice versa, but do not necessarily do so.

> ❗ It is important to identify whether it is only the channel that is disturbed or whether the internal organs are affected as well.

Channel pathologies arise for a variety of reasons:
• Invasion of external pathogenic factors
• Mechanical overexertion
• Traumas
• Transmitted disturbances in the viscera or bowels

To perform a correct channel diagnosis, close familiarity with their course is required.

6.8 Five Basic Substances Diagnosis

This theory assigns certain properties and functions to each of the basic substances *qi*, *xue*, *jin ye*, *shen*, and *jing*. Changes in any of these create defined pathological deviations. Overlaps with the theories of the eight principles and organ pathologies link these diagnostic systems.

One example of a disharmony in the area of the basic substances would be a lack of *jing*.

6.9 Five Elements Diagnosis

Every main channel is linked to its organ in a functional cycle. As a unit, they are associated with a phase, and in Chinese medicine, there are five phases: water, wood, fire, earth, and metal. These create a sequential cycle in this order. However, they also have the function of restraining and promoting each other, thereby ensuring a balanced equilibrium.

The diagnostic system of the five elements describes changes in the *sheng*/engendering cycle and the *ke*/restraining cycle. From this, the model of the *cheng*/overwhelming cycle and the *wu*/rebellion cycle results in which any imbalance between the phases disturbs the equilibrium in the body. One example of control according to the five phases would be if the phase of wood exerts excessive control over earth.

7 Acupuncture Points

The acupuncture points themselves are locations along the external channels where a higher number of nerve endings and capillaries cause resistance in the skin to be measurably lower. By stimulating these points, we are able to affect the flow of energy in the entire organism from here.

Up to now, roughly 400 points have been described in Traditional Chinese Veterinary Medicine (TCVM). In fact, however, the number is considerably higher. Acupuncture points can be summarized in groups. Depending on their correlation to the various diagnostic systems or the effects of points, they can achieve specific effects in different groups. An acupuncture point can hence appear in several groups and can be effective in a way that can be explained in the particular context of the underlying theory.

Correlations with the energy emission of various types of body cell and their bundling into standing waves in the meridian pathway currently offer convincing explanatory models for the effect of acupuncture points. Depending on the function or disturbance of the associated *zang* or *fu* organ, the energetic peak of the wave that forms the acupuncture point can easily move.

7.1 Transport Points

> The transport (*shu*) points are also called "ancient points" and form one of the most important groups of acupuncture points.

The term "transport point" refers here to its different abilities to transport *qi* and blood, pathogenic factors, warmth, cold, etc., along the course of the channel (▶ Table 7.1). The transport points lie distally on the extremities along the 12 main channels, on the standing animal from distal ascending to the height of the elbow or knee.

Progressing in a proximal direction, the property of *qi* changes sequentially from

Table 7.1 Transport points

Chinese name	English name	Effect I
Jing point	Well point	The most distal point where the *qi* emerges and flows very shallowly; the beginning or end point of the channel
Ying point	Brook point	Point that follows in a proximal direction where the *qi* accelerates; second point from the bottom
Shu point	Stream point	Point from where the flow of *qi* spreads out and moves more calmly; third point from the bottom
Jing point	River point	Point where the *qi* flows even more broadly and hence becomes more powerful and sustaining
He point	Sea point	Point where the *qi* flows into the depth; "*he*-sea located on elbow or knee"

one acupuncture point to the next. Its quality at the points can be compared with the changing flow properties of water from its spring to its mouth, as follows.

The Chinese term *jing* occurs twice, for well point and river point. The term *shu* also has a double meaning. On the one hand, it refers to the back transport *shu* points on the bladder channel; on the other hand, it refers to the ancient transport *shu* points. Because it is easy for misunderstandings to arise in the West if we use the Chinese names exclusively, combining them with the English names is a good option. Therefore, if we initially use the terms *jing*-well point and *jing*-river point, there are fewer opportunities for misunderstanding. The same holds true for the terms "ancient transport *shu* point" and "back transport *shu* point."

Each of the ancient points is furthermore associated with one of the five phases (see The Five Elements [Phases of Change] (p. 11)).

It is important to observe the principle that the quality of *qi* always changes with the flow of *qi* from distal to proximal. This corresponds to the direction of the *sheng* cycle of engendering in the five phases.

Nevertheless, a fundamental difference exists between the *yin* channels and the *yang* channels regarding the point localizations with the phases:
- *Yin* channel:
  - Most distal point (well point): wood transition point
  - Second most distal point (*ying* point): fire point (strongest *yang* properties)
- *Yang* channel:
  - Most distal point (well point): metal point
  - Second most distal point (*ying* transition point): water point (strongest *yin* properties)

At the second most distal point, a strong **yin–yang polarity** develops. The water point is located on the *yang* channels, having the strongest *yin* quality here. The fire point is located on the *yin* channels, with the strongest *yang* properties. One of the proposed explanations for this is that the polarity of *qi* switches at the well points and that a part of the quality of *qi* (i.e., *yin* or *yang*) from the previous channel continues to flow on into the new channel for a short distance. This manifests most clearly at the second most distal point. The quality of *qi* changes from distal to proximal in the order of the *sheng* cycle of engenderment in the five-phase theory (see ▸ Fig. 3.3).

Nevertheless, *qi* also flows:
- In the three hand *yin* channels (lung, heart, and pericardium channels) and in the three foot *yang* channels (bladder, gallbladder, and stomach channels) from proximal to distal.
- In the three hand *yang* channels (small intestine, triple burner, and large intestine channels) and in the three foot *yin* channels (spleen/pancreas, kidney, and liver channels) from distal to proximal.

Every channel transmits its energy to the following channel at the end points of the extremities. Thus, we are faced with two perspectives regarding the **flow of *qi* in the channels**:
1. Macrocosmic *qi* penetrates into the channels through the legs and then flows—widening like a river—in one direction into the body.
2. The body's own *qi* circulates in a continuous energy cycle from one channel to the next. In the human body, the *yang* channels run like the heavenly *yang qi* from above to below, that is, from the hands to the feet. The *yin* channels run from the feet upward, just like the *yin qi* of earth ascending through the feet (analogous to water rising through tree roots). This model has also been adopted in veterinary medicine.

7.2 Phase Points

 The term phase point refers to the five points on each main channel on the distal extremities that are each associated with one of the five phases.

- All *yang* channels start at the foreleg with the metal point and end at the hind leg with the metal point.
- All *yin* channels end at the foreleg with the wood point and begin at the hind leg with the wood point.

The sequence of the phase points corresponds to that of the *sheng* cycle. The points follow in order as if someone had cut off the *sheng*/engendering cycle at the respective *ting* point (see *Ting* Points (p. 44)) and then applied it along the leg toward the top. The phases follow each other and merge:

- On the *yin* channels, the wood, fire, and earth points (= spring points) follow each other from distal to proximal in direct numerical order.
- On the *yang* channels, the metal, water, wood, and spring points follow each other directly (according to numerical order).

A peculiarity of the gallbladder channel is that a point is inserted between water and wood. Other than that, the order of its phase points follows a mathematical sequence that makes localization easier:
GB-44/metal − 1 = GB-43/water
GB-43 − 2 = GB-41/wood
GB-41 − 3 = GB-38/fire
GB-38 − 4 = GB-34/earth

- All *yin* points on the tarsus and carpus are associated with **earth,** and all points on the elbow and knee with **water.**
- All *yang* points on the elbow and knee are associated with **earth.**

7.3 *Ting* Points

Ting points are the starting and ending points of the channels on the paws (► Fig. 7.1).

Points located here can be used, for example, as emergency points. From here, *qi* can be sent very quickly to the other end of the channel (► Table 7.2).

7.4 *Xi*-Cleft Points

At the *xi* or cleft points, *qi* and blood collect.

- *Xi* means crevice, tear, or opening. The points are well suited to the treatment of acute, painful processes. The cleft points on the *yin* channels additionally help in blood disorders. They are found between the toes and the elbows or knees (► Fig. 7.2).
- In addition to the 12 cleft points on the main channels (► Table 7.3), there are four additional cleft points on the extraordinary vessels (► Table 7.4). Thus, we have a total of 16 *xi* points.

7.5 Source Points

The source *qi* (*yuan qi*), which is "administered" by the triple burner, gathers at the source (*yuan*) points (► Table 7.5).

- On the *yin* channels, the source points are identical with the ancient transport points (as the third most distally lying points). They regulate as well as supplement the associated viscera.

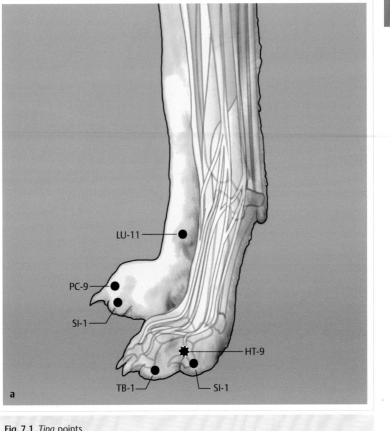

Fig. 7.1 *Ting* points.
a On the foreleg.

- On the *yang* channels, the source points are located between the transport and the well points (as the fourth most distally lying points, on the gallbladder channel as the fifth) and have no pronounced effect on their associated bowel. Rather, they remove excess pathogens from their channel.

- Besides their therapeutic effect, the source points can also be helpful in the diagnosis of disorders in the bowels because they respond to existing imbalances with sensitivity to pressure. Skin changes in this area can also indicate problems in the associated bowel.

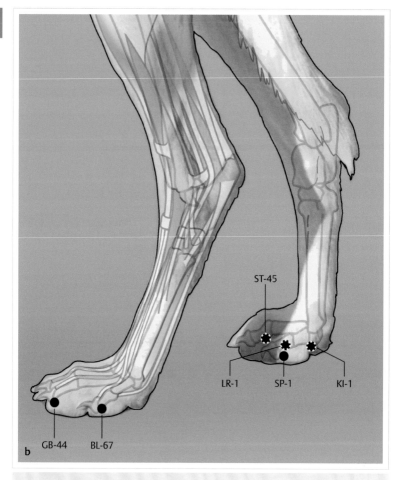

Fig. 7.1 (*Continued*) *Ting* points.
b On the hind leg.

While the *yin* source points thus supplement the viscera, the *yang* source points more effectively remove pathogenic factors in patterns of excess. Their strengthening effect on the bowels is therefore not their main task.

Table 7.2 *Ting* points and their localization

Ting point	Localization
Foreleg	
SI-1 (*yang* partner of HT-9)	Lateral on the 5th toe in *yang*
HT-9 (*yin* partner of SI-1)	Medial on the 5th toe in *yin*
TB-1	Lateral on the 4th (!) toe in *yang*
PC-9	Medial on the 3rd toe in *yang*
LU-11	Medial on the thumbnail of the 1st toe in *yin*
LI-1	Medial on the 2nd toe (near the lung *ting* point)
Hind leg	
SP-1	Medial on the 2nd toe; more plantar than LR-1 in *yin*
LR-1	Lateral on the 2nd toe
ST-45	Medial on the 3rd toe
KI-1	Between the 2nd and 3rd toes from below and from behind, needled under the large paw pad
BL-67	Lateral on the 5th toe in *yang*
GB-44	Lateral on the 4th toe in *yang*

7.6 Network Points

🛈 The network channels branch off at the network points of the 12 main channels. There are three additional network points: GV-1 of the governing vessel, CV-15 of the controlling vessel, and SP-21 of the spleen channel.

Thus, there are 15 network points (▶ Table 7.6). Applications of the network points are:

- Disorders of the *yin–yang* partner channels or the viscera and bowels
- Disorders in areas that are supplied by the network vessels
- Psychoemotional disorders

Network points are often used during treatment to bring *qi* into the coupled *yin* or *yang* channel. Parallel to this, you can needle the source point on the channel into which the *qi* is being directed (▶ Table 7.5).

7.7 Back Transport Points

🛈 Each main channel has its specific back transport point on the inner bladder channel to the left and right of the spinal column.

The 12 back transport points correspond to the viscera and bowels and lie on the inner bladder channel lateral to the midline (see ▶ Table 7.7 and ▶ **Fig. 7.3**; see Alternatives to Needle Acupuncture (p.62)). The name is composed of the associated viscus or bowel and the term *shu* (transport) point.

The transport points lie approximately at the level of the associated organ and are

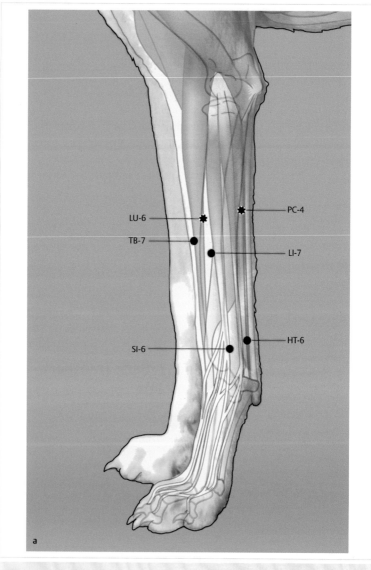

Fig. 7.2 *Xi*-cleft points.
a On the foreleg.

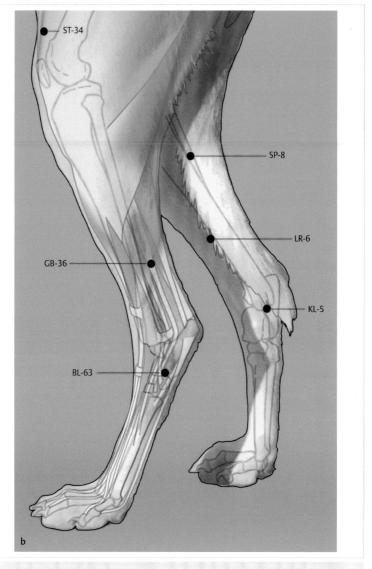

Fig. 7.2 (*Continued*) *Xi*-cleft points.
b On the hind leg.

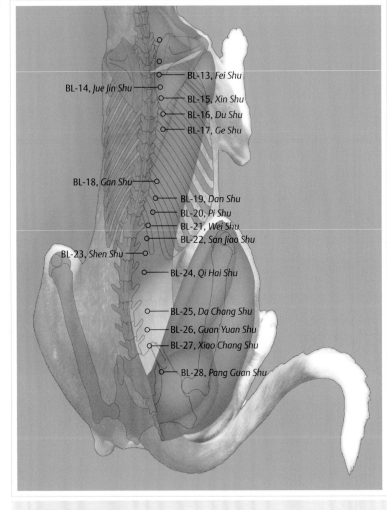

Fig. 7.3 Back *shu* points.

Table 7.3 Xi-cleft points of the 12 main channels on the foreleg and hind leg

Main channel	Xi-cleft point
Foreleg	
Lung	LU-6
Large intestine	LI-7
Heart	HT-6
Small intestine	SI-6
Triple burner	TB-7
Pericardium	PG4
Hind leg	
Stomach	ST-34
Spleen/pancreas	SP-8
Bladder	BL-63
Kidney	KI-5
Liver	LR-6
Gallbladder	GB-36

Table 7.5 Source points on the main channels

Main channel	Source point
Lung	LU-9
Large intestine	LI-4
Stomach	ST-42
Spleen/pancreas	SP-3
Heart	HT-7
Small intestine	SI-4
Bladder	BL-64
Kidney	KI-3
Pericardium	PG-7
Triple burner	TB-4
Gallbladder	GB-40
Liver	LR-3

Table 7.4 Xi-cleft points on the extraordinary vessels

Extraordinary vessel	Xi-cleft point
Yang qiao mai (yang springing vessel)	BL-59
Yin qiao mai (yin springing vessel)	KI-8
Yang wei mai (yang linking vessel)	GB-35
Yin wei mai (yin linking vessel)	KI-9

Table 7.6 Network points and their paired channels

Network point	Paired channel
LU-7	Large intestine
LI-6	Lung
ST-40	Spleen/pancreas
SP-4	Stomach
HT-5	Small intestine
S1-7	Heart
BL-58	Kidney
KI-4	Bladder
PC-6	Triple burner
TB-5	Pericardium
GB-37	Liver
LR-5	Gallbladder
CV-15	Governing vessel (du mai)
GV-1	Controlling vessel (ren mai)
SP-21	Connects all yin channels

Table 7.7 Back transport points

Transport point	Organ	Chinese name	Localization
BL-13	Lung	*Fei shu*	T3
BL-14	Pericardium	*Jue yin shu*	T4
BL-15	Heart	*Xin shu*	T5
BL-16*	Governing vessel	*Du shu*	T6
BL-17*	Diaphragm	*Ge shu*	T7
–	–	–	T8 + 9
BL-18	Liver	*Gan shu*	T10
BL-19	Gallbladder	*Dan shu*	T11
BL-20	Spleen	*Pi shu*	T12
BL-21	Stomach	*Wei shu*	T13
BL-22	Triple burner	*San jiao shu*	L1
BL-23	Kidney	*Shen shu*	L2
BL-24*	*Qi hai*	*Qi hai shu*	L3
–	–	–	L4
BL-25	Large intestine	*Da chang shu*	L5
BL-26*	*Guan yuan*	*Guan yuan shu*	L6
BL-27	Small intestine	*Xiao chang shu*	L7
BL-28	Bladder	*Pang guan shu*	Sacral foramen

* Classical transport points that are not associated with the main channels.

extremely useful in diagnosis because they become sensitive to pressure when the relevant functional cycle is in a state of imbalance. In this context, patients with an existing problem of excess respond with pain to minor pressure, whereas they are more likely to react to stronger stimulation in deficiency conditions.

In addition to the points that are associated with the 12 main channels and functional cycles, there are additional classical transport points (▶ Table 7.7).

Some of these also find clinical application in veterinary medicine, whether for diagnosis or for treatment.

According to the classical texts, the back transport points are more suitable for treating deficiency and cold in the viscera than problems in the bowels because the points are located in *yang*, and therefore treat *yin* disorders most effectively. *Yang*, here, treats *yin*.

The bowels are better treated by means of the alarm (*mu*) points, which lie in *yin*. Here, *yin* treats *yang*.

7.8 Alarm Points

The 12 alarm (*mu*) points are located on the abdomen or thorax in the vicinity of the associated organ.

Each viscus or bowel also has its "own" alarm point. The *qi* of the viscera and bowels collects and concentrates in the alarm points. In disorders of their associated viscus or bowel, alarm and transport points easily become sensitive to pressure. The sensitivity of the alarm points gives a clear indication of the potential involvement of the organ in the presenting pathology (▶ Table 7.8).

Only the alarm points of the lung (LU-1), liver (LR-14), and gallbladder (GB-24) lie on their own channel. Six additional alarm points lie on the controlling vessel (*ren mai*).

A mnemonic device for memorizing the sequence of the alarm points is: Triple burner (CV-5), small intestine (CV-4), bladder (CV-3): **TSB—three small boys.**

Table 7.8 Alarm points

Alarm point	Organ
LU-1	Lung
ST-25	Large intestine
CV-12	Stomach
LR-13	Spleen/pancreas
CV-14	Heart
CV-4	Small intestine
CV-3	Bladder
GB-25	Kidney
CV-17	Pericardium
CV-5	Triple burner
GB-24	Gallbladder
LR-14	Liver

7.9 Meeting Points

The eight meeting (*hui*) points are often called "influential points" or "master points of the types of tissues."

The effect of the meeting points (▶ Table 7.9) on certain body tissues is particularly great, and they are needled in order to support the associated tissue.

Table 7.9 Meeting points

Meeting point	Effect
LR-13 (*pi mu*)	Master point of the viscera and of the body as a whole
CV-12 (*wei mu*)	Affects all bowels
CV-17 (*xin bao mu*)	Sea of *qi*, influences especially the *zong qi*
BL-17 (*ge shu*)	Master point of the blood (treats all forms of blood heat, deficiency, and stasis)
GB-34	Master point of the tendons in the entire body (especially for contractions and stiffness)
LU-9	Master point of the pulse and blood vessels (especially for bloody cough or vomiting of blood, and blood stasis in the heart and thorax due to weakness of *zong* [ancestral] *qi*)
BL-11	Influential point of the bones (for painful deformations of the bones and stiffness and pain in the spinal column, neck, and lumbar region)
GB-39	Master point of the marrow (for strengthening tendons and bones, has broad applicability in the context of weakness, deficiency, flaccidity, and contraction of the extremities)

Table 7.10 Master points of the body regions

Master point	Body region
LI-4	Head, muzzle, and face
LU-7	Nape, neck, and occipital area
ST-36	Stomach area
BL-40	Back and lumbar area
PC-6	Thorax

Table 7.11 Lower sea points and associated bowels

Point	Bowel
ST-37	Large intestine
ST-39	Small intestine
BL-39	Triple burner

Table 7.12 Four seas points

Sea	Points	Application
Sea of *qi*	ST-9, CV-17, GV-15, GV-14	For excess/deficiency
Sea of blood	Thoroughfare vessel (*chong mai*) BL-11, ST-37, ST-39	Jointly for supplementation, (e.g., for blood deficiency)
Sea of water and of grain	ST-30 (upper point) ST-36 (lower point)	Excess causes a feeling of fullness; deficiency causes hunger with inability to eat
Sea of marrow	GV-20 (upper point) GV-16 (lower point)	Improves brain activity

7.10 Master Points of the Body Regions

The master points are empirically discovered points with a special effect on certain body regions.

The master points (▶ Table 7.10) can reinforce the effect of local points or specific points on a particular region.

7.11 Lower Sea Points

The lower sea points (*he* points) have a stronger effect on the associated bowels than the "regular" sea points of the ancient

transport point system, which are located on the relevant channel itself (▶ Table 7.11).

7.12 Points of the Four Seas

The text *"Spiritual Pivot"* (*Ling Shu*) describes four seas in the body (▶ Table 7.12). These are point combinations that have a specific targeted effect on the *qi*, blood, nutrition, or marrow, and intervene here by regulation.

Suggested Reading

Zhang C. Der unsichtbare Regenbogen und die unhörbare Musik. Traumzeit Verlag; 2010

8 Point Selection

There are numerous theories on point selection. In this book, we present a brief overview. Only a well-founded education in acupuncture can convey the necessary professional expertise.

Clear differences in point selection can arise between the different theories, and seeming contradictions can cause irritation. Some people feel safer with the consistent application of a single theory, while others are happy with a large spectrum of options and variations in the treatment of a great diversity of patients. It certainly makes sense to become well acquainted with the various systems, so that you are able to choose the best therapy in any individual case. For greatest expediency, we should be thoroughly familiar with the effects of individual points on the different combinable channels as well as in different contexts, and to match them as effectively as possible. We should ask ourselves again and again: What is the problem? What do I want to effect? Which points can achieve this goal?

As a rule, acupuncture treatment should balance the energy in the body and thereby restore its equilibrium. The selection of acupuncture points for therapy must therefore always correspond to the applied diagnostic system.

Ah Shi Points Needling pressure-sensitive points (*ah shi* points) is the easiest treatment method. For this purpose, palpate a sensitive point such as a muscle and needle it directly to achieve a localized relaxation. The pain-relieving, anticonvulsant, local effect is of primary importance.

Transport Points Needling pressure-sensitive transport points has a simultaneous effect on the associated organ. According to the classical texts, the back transport points are more suitable for treating deficiency and cold in the viscera than problems in the bowels. This is because the points are located in *yang* and therefore treat *yin* disorders most effectively. *Yang*, here, treats *yin*.

The bowels are better treated by means of the alarm points, which lie in *yin*. Here, *yin* treats *yang*.

Organ Pathology When we diagnose a pathology of the viscera or bowels (e.g., kidney *yang* deficiency), we must orient the acupuncture treatment toward it. The selected points are chosen based on the affected channel or functional cycle and their specific effect.

We cannot correct a blood deficiency by only expelling wind. Even when the animal presents with itching as the primary symptom caused by the blood deficiency, we must make it our priority to remove the underlying symptom; namely, the blood deficiency. We cannot treat a kidney *yang* deficiency by expelling dampness, but have to select a point such as KI-7 that strengthens kidney *yang*. Liver *qi* stagnation, for example, is treated by moving *qi* and blood in the liver channel. For this purpose, the combination LR-3/LR-2 is highly effective.

Five-Phase Theory When selecting points based on the five-phase theory, according to which the channels nurture and restrain each other, we observe the energetic relationship between the channels and strive for an equilibrium. If metal is too weak to restrain wood and wood therefore suffers from pathological excess, therapy aims at strengthening the lung channel, to regain control. This would be possible, for example, by needling the supplementing point (LU-9, earth) on the lung channel.

Ancient Transport Points   When using the ancient transport points, our focus lies with the different quality of *qi* at the relevant location. At the most distal point, for example, one can reach *qi* that is rapidly flowing into the channel. Near the trunk, by contrast, at the *he*-sea points, we address *qi* that has direct influence on the associated organs.

Network–Source Combination Points
The combination of network points and source points creates a balance between the partnered *yin* and *yang* channels in a functional cycle. Here, we first needle the network point of the partner channel that has more *qi*. The *qi* then emerges at the source point on the partner channel, which is needled next, and flows into that channel. By this method, we can strengthen the weaker channel. A prerequisite for this method is an energetic imbalance between the *yin* and *yang* partner channels. There has to be enough *qi* present in the channel on which the network point is needled to achieve an effect.

Master Points   We needle master points to treat a specific diseased tissue or affected body region.

Organ Clock   In selecting points according to the organ clock, we consider the occurrence of symptoms at specific times of the day.

Xi-cleft Points   These points are used to treat acute painful and/or bleeding p/or bleeding processes by needling the channel associated with the affected organ/functional cycle or tissue.

9 Point Identification and Needling

One common gradation of the distances between points is done by means of the Chinese measurement cun. In dogs and cats, 1 cun corresponds to the width of the patient's calcaneus (▶ Fig. 9.1).

The **detection** of acupuncture points primarily takes its cue from anatomical descriptions and is done by palpation. Nevertheless, it is important to know that acupuncture in ancient China rarely worked with exact point descriptions. For that era, it would be more accurate to speak of reactive areas than precise points. Even today, acupuncturists are well advised to test the reactivity of an acupuncture point at the described location before needling it. To touch, palpate, and feel where the correct point is located is, and remains, an important aspect of acupuncture. Feelings of cold or warmth, tingling, etc., are possible sensations that the acupuncturist will experience with the finger at the reactive acupuncture point.

A point should always be needled only after palpation. It can be helpful to place one finger next to the point during needling, to tighten the tissue for easier needle insertion and to use the finger pressure to distract from the prick.

The particular **direction of insertion** depends on the underlying structure. A tangential (almost parallel to the body's surface) or oblique (approximately 45 degrees caudal or distal) direction of insertion can be helpful to prevent the needle from slipping out and to spare, for example, underlying joints, nerves, or blood vessels (▶ Fig. 9.2).

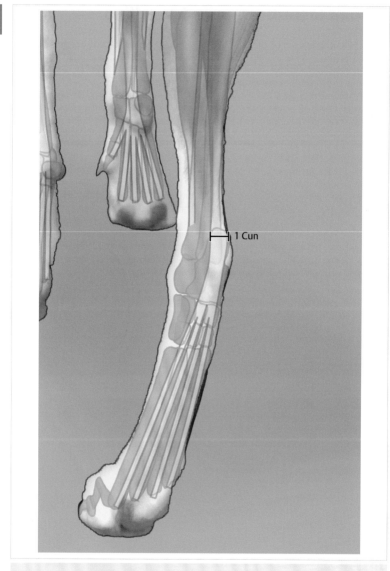

Fig. 9.1 The width of the patient's calcaneus corresponds to 1 cun.

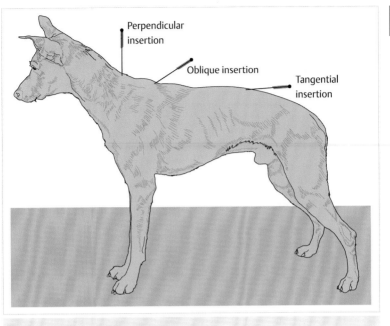

Fig. 9.2 Vertical, tangential, and oblique needling.

10 Forms of Acupuncture

10.1 Acupuncture Needles

In veterinary acupuncture, we use fine, elastic, sterile disposable needles from human medicine. Steel needles are one option, but we also use needles made from gold and silver. There are silicone-coated needles as well as uncoated needles. The coating allows the fine needles to penetrate the skin more easily and with less pain, but can also cause them to slip out more quickly if the patient moves while the needles are in place.

Acupuncture needles available commercially are tested for quality assurance and are generally quite safe. In spite of this, practitioners should be aware of their responsibility for the patient and always examine the condition of the needles for safety. Only use needles that are packaged and sterile. Packages that have been opened for an extended period of time or damaged are no longer sterile, and can present a risk of infection.

Disposable needles are for one-time use only. If reused, they would, aside from the problem of hygiene, become dull and therefore penetrate less easily into tissue.

10.1.1 Needle Types

In general, you can choose between two needle types: the Hwato and the Seirin types.

Hwato Needles These needles are less sharp at the tip and have flexible coiled metal handles. Hence, they are somewhat more difficult to push through the skin. On the other hand, they are better at conducting electricity and warmth and are therefore particularly suitable for moxibustion and electro-acupuncture.

Seirin Needles These are sharper and have hard plastic handles, facilitating a quick, painless insertion.

For small animals, it is best to use needles of 0.20×15 mm, 0.30×30 mm, and 0.35×50 mm. Small needles (0.20×15 mm) are used mostly on the head, thorax, and distal extremities, while larger needles (0.30×30 mm or more) are required for areas with thicker muscle mass.

The longer and thinner a needle, the more difficult it is to insert. The use of injection cannulas for acupuncture entails risks and should therefore be avoided. In acupuncture, the needles remain in the tissue for some time before they are removed. Injection cannulas are stiff, and as a result they can easily damage the tissue when the patient moves, and are more likely to break under strain. Furthermore, they have a lumen, which increases the risk of infiltration of contaminants.

In human acupuncture, we also see needles used with small tubes. This is impractical in veterinary medicine because one first has to position and apply the tube in preparation for the insertion, something that experience has shown not to be tolerated well by dogs and cats. They can react to this preparation with irritation and rejection.

The least irritation is caused by direct, quick insertion, potentially supported by pressure with one finger in the vicinity of the acupuncture point that one is about to needle.

10.1.2 Acupuncture in Small Animals

Acupuncture must always be implemented with expert knowledge and caution. Thus, the following should be noted.

- Monitor the patient's general state of health and circulatory condition.
- In case of a severe and persistent pain response, check for the correct location of a needle and, if necessary, remove it. Several seconds after insertion, the patient should be able to tolerate the applied needles well. Strong pain is not helpful for the effect of the acupuncture treatment and should be avoided. The desired sensation of *de qi* (see *De Qi*) is nothing but a faint twitch or a feeling of pressure.
- Tingling, a feeling of pressure, or a sensation of warmth, which causes the animal to try and pull out the needle, should be reduced by distracting or holding the patient.
- While the needles stay in, the patient must be monitored at all times to keep the animal from swallowing a needle by licking or nibbling it off.
- An additional risk is acupuncture in the vicinity of joints. Never insert an acupuncture needle into a joint. Serious tissue damage and joint infections can be the dire consequences.
- Special caution is also required in the area of the thorax. Inserting the needle too deeply can cause a pneumothorax. The same holds true for the back transport points in this area.
- Avoid damaging blood vessels and nerve tissue.
- In the area of the lower abdomen, there is a risk of accidentally puncturing the urinary bladder if it is very full. Other abdominal organs, especially when they are enlarged, can also be injured with a needle that is too long.

De Qi To achieve a therapeutic effect, acupuncture has to set energies in motion. This effect expresses itself, for example, in a sensation of tingling along the affected channels, a feeling like an electrical current, in a sensation of pressure at the needled point, or in a feeling of warmth in the tissue.

As a practitioner, the desired *de qi* effect you want to reach during treatment feels as if the tissue is grasping the needle. If you get the feeling of poking around in an empty space, you have not reached *de qi*. In this case, it can be helpful to gently raise and lower the needle or to rotate it. It is also possible that you will have to adjust the position of the needle.

10.1.3 Needling Techniques

There are several possibilities in needling for sedation or tonification. Here, the practitioner must take the patient's physical condition into consideration (▶ Table 10.1).

These possibilities are not to be confused with the tonification and sedation points on the lower extremities. These are connected to the five-phase cycles, where each phase is nourished by the preceding mother phase and passes energy on to the following child phase.

Each channel has five phase points. Hence, there is one tonification and one

Table 10.1 Possibilities of tonifying and sedating needling

	Tonifying	Sedating
Needle insertion	Slow	Quick
Needle removal	Quick → *qi* is not pulled out along with the needle	Slow → *qi* is pulled out of the body
Length of needle retention	10–20 minutes	20–30 minutes
Needle rotation	In a clockwise direction	In a counterclockwise direction

sedation point for each. The tonification point is that phase point within the engendering cycle that comes before the particular phase point (wood point on the wood channel, water point on the water channel, etc.) on the affected channel. The sedation point is the point that follows after the particular phase point.

10.2 Alternatives to Needle Acupuncture

Hemoacupuncture To remove pathogenic *qi* from a channel, there is the option of bleeding acupuncture points.

Aquapuncture We can use injection cannulas to inject fluids into acupuncture points. The slow absorption of fluid in the tissue creates longer-lasting pressure at the acupuncture point, which is meant to amplify the effect of the needle. Injectable substances are, among others, Traumeel (Heel, Baden-Baden, Germany), echinacea, vitamin B_{12}, or anesthetics such as lidocaine.

Moxibustion Moxa is produced from *Artemisia vulgaris* (mugwort) and is used in different forms. In veterinary medicine, the preferred form is pressed moxa cigars, with or without smoke development, or loose moxa. During application, moxa is lit and develops a very particular aromatic fragrance and a very special heat quality. This property activates *yang* and disperses cold and dampness. The smell penetrates into the channels, to move *qi* and blood there. Moxa is effective for conditions such as cold and *qi* stagnation in the channels, painful joints, numbness, infertility, and paralysis. For dogs and cats, it is easiest to light moxa in cigar form and then hold it or wave it back and forth at a distance of approximately 2 cm above the relevant acupuncture point. With the other hand,

check the developing heat. Moxa easily brings energy into the body. The application of moxa is contraindicated during pregnancy and in inflammatory processes.

Laser Acupuncture Lasers are used to stimulate body cells or acupuncture points with light energy. Laser acupuncture is painless and therefore bearable even for patients with needle phobia. Different frequencies cause specific effects. Training in the use of a laser device is recommended to avoid risks related to the application of laser light.

Electrostimulation By attaching the ends of small charged wires to inserted acupuncture needles, we can conduct electricity and hence *yang* energy into the acupuncture points.

Especially for treating *wei* syndrome, herniated disk, paralyses, or other neurological deficits, it is very helpful to support acupuncture with electricity. This is, however, contraindicated in pregnancy, with epilepsy, and with cardiovascular problems.

Most devices have four outputs for two wires each. The current can be regulated for each pair. The number of current pulses per minute is adjusted with the frequency. Here, it is best to use a varying frequency (intermittent) or a dispense/disperse mode with changing intensity and set intervals, so that the body is unable to adapt to the current and thereby lose its response to the stimulus. In A/C mode, the device operates with an alternating current; in D/C mode, the direct current flows from the negative to the positive electrode.

Gold Acupuncture or Gold Implantation This method is applied most commonly to achieve a permanent effect and improvement in chronic degenerative joint disease.

For a permanent effect, we can implant gold wires or balls into the acupuncture points. To implant the gold safely, the surgery must be performed under sterile operating conditions and under anesthesia. The implants must be placed precisely, and after a thorough examination of the individual case, to achieve the best effect possible.

Ideally, in gold acupuncture, the gold is placed purposely on those acupuncture points that balance the entire organism and have a delineated effect on the affected joint problem. The random insertion of implants in the vicinity of the joint might produce improvement "by coincidence," but can possibly also cause undesired results that will only manifest later and may never be associated with the implantation.

Potential complications can be postoperative infections, penetration of the joint capsule, and nerve irritations.

The most common indications include hip dysplasia, elbow arthrosis, gonarthrosis, and spondylosis.

Sound Acupuncture Sound acupuncture utilizes the vibrations transmitted to acupuncture points via tuning forks at different tuning levels, with which the points resonate. The functional cycles and channels are associated with specific frequencies and are thus stimulated by sound accordingly.

Crystal Acupuncture Crystal rods are mostly used in accordance with their specific properties and mode of action. This effect is amplified by the use of corresponding acupuncture points. The effects of the crystals are produced by their structure and composition.

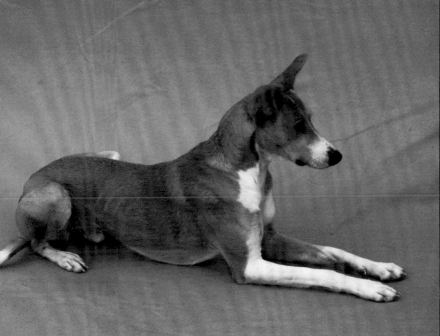

II Atlas of Acupuncture Points

11 Lung Channel

Hand *Tai Yin* (*Shou Tai Yin Fei Mai* 手太阴肺脉)

Originating in the middle burner in the stomach area, one branch of the lung channel runs downward to the large intestine, another branch runs across the mouth of the cardia, through the diaphragm into the lungs, and from there into the throat. Here, it turns around and runs back down, to come to the surface at the point LU-1 in the first intercostal space. From there, it runs below the surface of the body along the inside of the foreleg in a distal direction to the medial nail fold of the first toe. At the point LU-7, a small branch separates off to link up with the large intestine channel at LI-1 on the second toe.

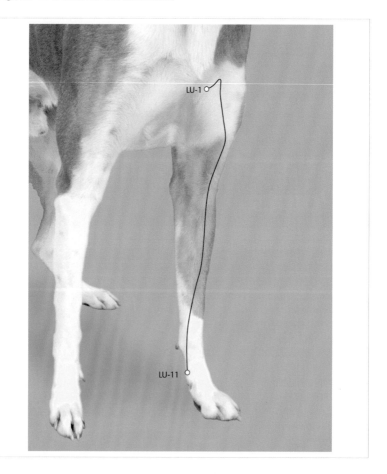

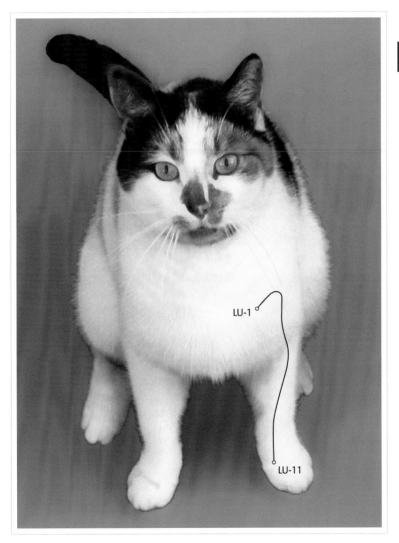

LU

LU-1 Central Treasury

中府 *Zhong Fu*

Mu-alarm point, intersection point with the spleen channel.

Effect Stimulates the descent of lung *qi*, disperses fullness and phlegm in the chest area, regulates the waterways, brings down stomach *qi*.

Indications Respiratory health problems, bronchitis, asthma, painful itchy dermatoses, localized problems in the areas of the shoulder and chest, swelling of the shoulder joint. In conjunction with LR-14, this point resolves stagnation that led to a raging lack of self-worth due to isolation from heavenly inspiration.

Localization First intercostal space, medial to the major tubercle of the humerus, in the superficial and descending pectoral muscle.

Technique To a depth of about 0.3 cun; perpendicular insertion.

 Jugular trunk; do not needle in the direction of the thorax wall as there is a risk of pneumothorax.

LU-2 Cloud Gate

云门 *Yun Men*

Effect Promotes the descent of lung *qi*, clears lung heat.

Indications Respiratory health problems, bronchitis, asthma, painful localized problems in the area of the shoulder and chest, swelling of the shoulder joint, and a loss of instinct due to a lack of grounding. Overall a weaker effect than LU-1.

Localization In the first intercostal space, medial to the major tubercle of the humerus, slightly closer to it and above LU-1.

Technique To a depth of about 0.3 cun; perpendicular insertion.

 Jugular trunk; do not needle in the direction of the thorax wall as there is a risk of pneumothorax.

LU-3 Celestial Storehouse

天府 *Tian Fu*

Effect Brings down lung *qi*, clears lung heat, cools blood, stanches bleeding, calms the corporeal (*po*) soul.

Indications Pain on the inside of the upper arm, shoulder pain, labored breathing, asthma. For claustrophobia, regulates excessive neediness in hand-raised animals.

Localization Inside by the beginning of the upper third of the humerus on the lateral edge of the biceps muscle of the arm at the height of the terminal tendons of the pectoral muscles.

Technique To a depth of about 0.5 cun; perpendicular insertion.

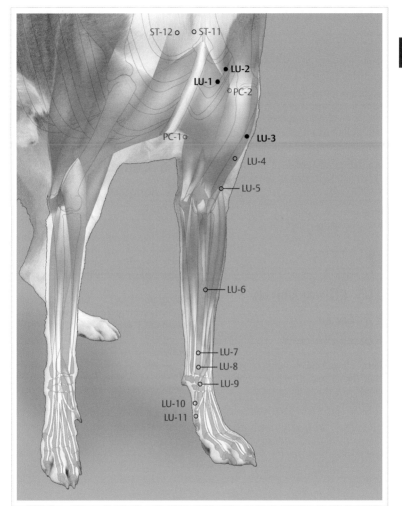

ST-12 ○ ○ ST-11

LU

● LU-2

LU-1 ●

○ PC-2

PC-1 ○   ● LU-3

○ LU-4

○ LU-5

○ LU-6

○ LU-7

○ LU-8

○ LU-9

LU-10 ○

LU-11 ○

LU

LU-4 Guarding White

侠白 *Xia Bai*

Effect Regulates *qi* and blood in the thorax, brings down lung *qi*.

Indications Pain on the inside of the arm and in the thorax, which can lead to problems with bringing the extremities forward, dyspnea, cough. Strengthens in cases of overwork that leads to isolation.

Localization Craniolateral in the center of the humerus, lateral to the biceps muscle of the arm.

Technique To a depth of about 0.3 cun; perpendicular insertion.

 Cephalic vein

LU-5 Elbow Marsh

尺泽 *Chi Ze*

He-sea point, water point.

Effect Clears lung heat and phlegm, stimulates the descent of lung *qi*, supports the bladder by opening the waterways, relaxes the tendons.

Indications Respiratory problems with phlegm production, asthma, pulmonary emphysema, pain in the elbow joint, weakness of the foreleg, urinary retention, eczema in the flews, nasal pyoderma, edemas. Restores movement in rigid behavioral patterns.

Localization Medial in the elbow fold, between the brachial muscle and the biceps tendon.

Technique To a depth of about 0.3 cun; perpendicular insertion.

LU-6 Collection Hole

孔最 *Kong Zui*

Xi-cleft point.

Effect Harmonizes and brings down lung *qi*, clears heat and moistens the lung, stanches bleeding, mobilizes reserves, discharges pathological fullness.

Indications Pain in the foreleg with impaired mobility, asthma, laryngitis, acute pneumonia. Helps with accepting grief.

Localization In the upper third of the radius, in the middle of the distance between LU-5 and LU-7, medial to the extensor carpi radialis muscle.

Technique To a depth of about 0.5 cun; perpendicular insertion.

LU

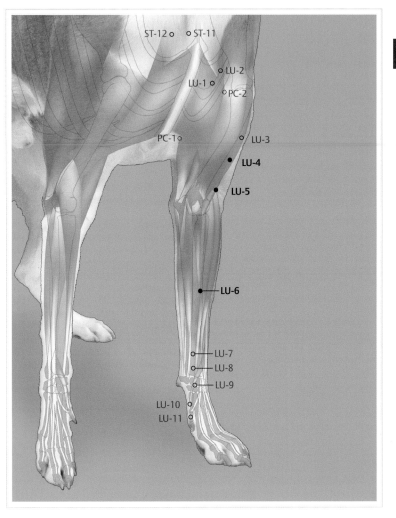

LU

LU-7 Broken Sequence

列缺 *Lie Que*

Luo-network point, master point for the head and nape, opener of the controlling vessel (*ren mai*), partner point of the *yin qiao mai* (*yin* springing vessel).

Effect Expels external wind; stimulates defense (*wei*) *qi*; stimulates the descent and distribution of lung *qi*; moves phlegm; opens the pores, nose, and waterways, better suited for lung repletion patterns; supports the head and nape.

Indications Any problem with the neck and nape, asthma and any kind of cough, acute or chronic inflammation of the upper respiratory tracts and associated anorexia, localized problems of the carpal joint, facial nerve paresis, trigeminal neuralgia, weakness, urinary retention, obstipation, chronic diarrhea, edema in the shoulder and joints of the foreleg. Releases deep-seated grief. In conjunction with LI-6, it invigorates circulation between the *yin* and *yang* aspects of metal. Promotes mental agility. In a row with LU-1 to -7 to LI-4 to -20, it restores the intake-and-discharge process.

Localization Proximal to the styloid process of the radius, 1.5 cun above the carpal flexion crease, distal to the point where the accessory cephalic vein branches off from the cephalic vein.

Technique To a depth of about 0.5 cun; oblique insertion in a distal direction.

LU-8 Channel Ditch

经渠 *Jing Qu*

Jing-river point, metal point.

Effect Brings down lung *qi*, relieves coughing and panting.

Indications Cough, asthma, pain in the elbow and carpal joint. Clears inadequately processed experiences, helps to release the old in order to experience the new.

Localization At the height of the medial styloid process, directly on the radial artery and the tendon of the flexor carpi radialis muscle.

Technique To a depth of about 0.2 cun; oblique insertion in a distal direction.

 Radial artery

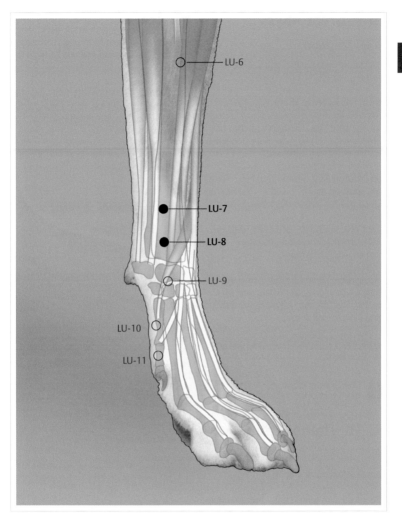

LU-6

LU-7

LU-8

LU-9

LU-10

LU-11

LU

LU-9 Great Abyss

太渊 *Tai Yuan*

Shu-stream point, earth and source point, master point for the blood vessels.

Effect Transforms phlegm; supplements lung *qi* and *yin*; influences blood circulation, the blood vessels, and the pulse; compared with LU-7, it is used more frequently for lung deficiency patterns.

Indications Respiratory problems; cough with sputum; asthma; pain in the chest, in the carpus, or inside the foreleg; circulatory disorders; vascular disorders; compared with LU-7, it is used more frequently for internal deficiency disorders. Frees from addictive behaviors.

Localization Distal to the medial styloid process and the radial carpal bone, on the medial end of the carpal joint crease, medial to the radial artery.

Technique To a depth of about 0.2 cun; oblique insertion in a distal direction.

❗ Joint gap and radial artery

LU-10 Thenar Eminence

鱼际 *Yu Ji*

Ying-brook point, fire point.

Effect Clears lung heat, brings down rebellious lung *qi*, supports the throat, harmonizes the heart and stomach.

Indications Lung disease with fever, cough, pharyngitis, pain in the neck, shoulder, elbow, and entire foreleg. It dissolves rejecting distance and stiffness through fire energy.

Localization Between the first and second metacarpal bones, seen from palmar in the middle of the length of the first metacarpal bone.

Technique To a depth of about 0.3 cun; perpendicular insertion.

LU-11 Lesser *Shang*

少商 *Shao Shang*

Jing-well point, wood point.

Effect Clears heat and wind, supports the throat, stimulates the descent of lung *qi*, restores consciousness.

Indications Arthralgia in the toe joints of the foreleg, inflammation and pain in the throat area, epistaxis, sinusitis, bronchitis, esophageal spasms, fever, manifested grief. Dispels wind in convulsive fits that are associated with fear. Wood aggression due to lung deficiency/grief/loss.

Localization Medial claw fold of the first toe of the front paw.

Technique To a depth of about 0.2 cun; oblique insertion in a distal direction.

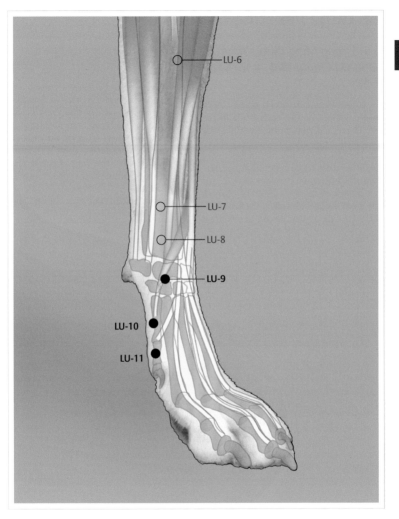

12 Large Intestine Channel

Hand *Yang Ming* (*Shou Yang Ming Da Chang Mai* 手阳明大肠脉)

The large intestine channel begins medially on the forefoot on the medial side of the second toe and runs mediodorsally along the limb in a proximal direction to the carpus. Here it crosses over and moves to the dorsolateral aspect, to continue dorsolaterally to the elbow and shoulder joint.

A branch of the large intestine channel runs from the shoulder along the ventrolateral side of the throat upward to penetrate through the cheek directly into the gums of the lower jaw. From the gums, the channel continues across the cheek to the point LI-20, where it ends. Whether it crosses over to the other side of the body, as described in the human body, is under discussion. From the shoulder, one branch runs to the point GV-14, where it meets up with the other five *yang* channels. There it connects deep down with the lung before it runs through the diaphragm to connect with the large intestine.

Another branch runs from the shoulder down to the point ST-37.

LI

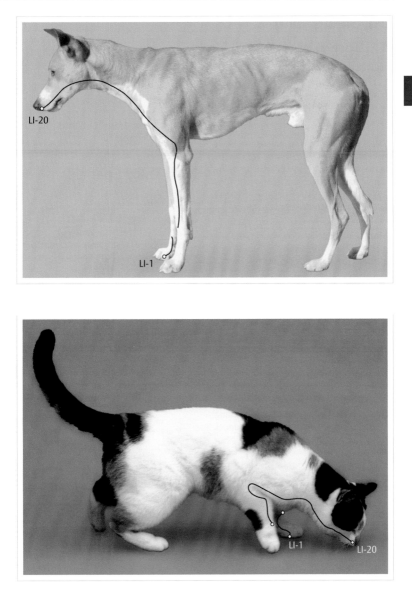

LI-1 Shang Yang

商阳 *Shang Yang*

Jing-well point, metal point.

Effect Dispels heat and swellings, clears the eyes, restores consciousness, moves *qi* along the channel.

Indications Acute, possibly febrile, laryngitis; pharyngitis; tonsillitis; toothache; circulatory collapse; shoulder pain; elbow pain; arthrosis of the toe joint in the front paw. Clears patterns of negative expectations due to unprocessed grief.

Localization Medial claw fold on the second toe of the front paw.

Technique To a depth of about 0.2 cun; oblique insertion in a proximal direction.

LI-2 Second Space

二间 *Er Jian*

Ying-brook point, water point, sedation point.

Effect Dispels wind, heat, and swelling; clears the eyes; moves *qi* along the channel.

Indications Acute, possibly febrile, laryngitis; pharyngitis; tonsillitis; toothache; circulatory collapse. Softens internal rigidity.

Localization Medial on the base of the second fore toe just below the metacarpal joint between the proximal and distal phalanges.

Technique To a depth of about 0.2 cun; perpendicular insertion.

LI-3 Third Space

三间 *San Jian*

Shu-stream point, wood point.

Effect Dispels wind, heat, and repletion; clears heat; supports the eyes, throat, and teeth.

Indications Pain and spasms in the paw; shoulder pain; facial nerve paresis; inflammation of the eyes, throat, and ears; toothache; inflammation of the skin and mucosa. Helps with the processing of traumas when these are triggered.

Localization Medial on the base of the second fore toe just above the metacarpal joint between the proximal and distal phalanges.

Technique To a depth of about 0.2 cun; perpendicular insertion.

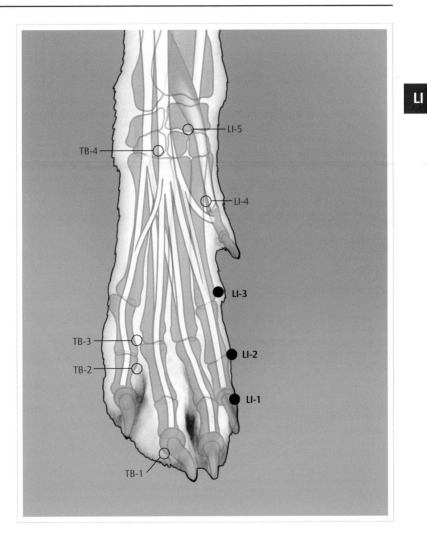

LI

LI-4 Union Valley
合谷 *He Gu*

Yuan-source point, master point for the head and mouth.

Effect Dispels wind heat, frees the surface, regulates defense (*wei*) *qi*, resolves obstructions in the channel, stimulates the distribution function of the lung, regulates the face.

Indications Any problem related to the face and mouth, toothache, rhinitis, sinusitis, laryngopharyngitis, facial nerve paresis, trigeminal neuralgia, immune stimulation, dermatitis with itching, very important for sedation, fever, problems in the large intestine and lung, weakness at birth, distal point for any channel problem but especially on the foreleg and nape, local problems of the fore toe and carpus, important for acupuncture analgesia. As the great discharger, it helps to get rid of rigid posture or fixed grief. In conjunction with LR-3, the "four gates" calm down a hyper-nervous disposition. LI-4 + CV-3, CV-24, and GB-13 calm the soul.

Localization Between the first and second metacarpal bones, at the level of the middle of the second phalanx of the first toe
in the front paw. Alternatively, LI-4 is described as being located between the second and third metacarpal bones, approximately at the height of their center.

Technique To a depth of about 0.3 cun; perpendicular insertion.

 Contraindicated during pregnancy.

LI-5 *Yang* Ravine
阳溪 *Yang Xi*

Jing-river point, fire point.

Effect Clears heat, calms the spirit, moves *qi* along the channel, strengthens the carpal joint.

Indications Toothache, pain in the carpal joint, pain and inflammation of the eyes and eyelids, itching. Clears bizarre behavior patterns that are due to the effect of heat.

Localization Distal and slightly dorsal to the medial styloid process on the carpal joint.

Technique To a depth of about 0.3 cun; perpendicular insertion.

LI-6 Veering Passageway
偏历 *Pian Li*

Luo-network point.

Effect Eliminates wind, clears heat, opens the waterways of the lung.

Indications Pain in the shoulder, forearm, and carpal joint, ascites, toothache, sore throat, facial nerve paresis. Helps to realize losses.

Localization Craniomedial in the lower third of the length of the radius, at the level of the point where the accessory cephalic vein branches off from the cephalic vein.

Technique To a depth of about 0.3 cun; perpendicular insertion.

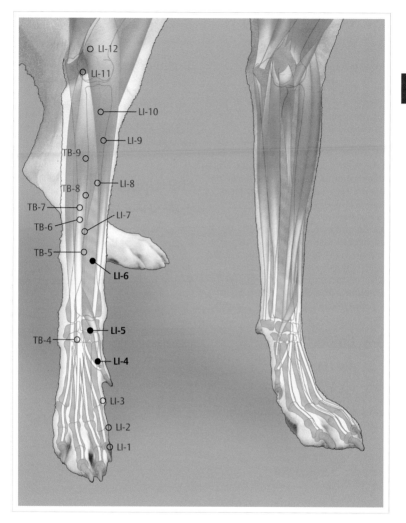

LI

LI-7 Warm Dwelling

温溜 *Wen Liu*

Xi-cleft point.

Effect Clears heat and fire in the large intestine and stomach channels of *yang ming*, removes toxins, regulates the stomach and intestines, calms the spirit.

Indications Acute pain and inflammation in the foreleg, carpal joint problems, acute inflammation in the area of the throat and pharynx. For attachment to old patterns.

Localization Between the tendons of the extensor carpi radialis and extensor digitorum muscles, laterodorsal on the transition from the lower to the middle third of the length of the shank of the foreleg.

Technique To a depth of about 0.3 cun; perpendicular insertion.

LI-8 Lower Ridge

下廉 *Xia Lian*

Effect Dispels wind-heat, clears fire in the large intestine and stomach *yang ming* channels, calms the spirit, harmonizes the large intestine.

Indications Pain in the shoulder and foreleg, carpal joint pain, edemas, painful diarrhea.

Localization Just above the half of the length of the forearm, between the extensor carpi radialis and the extensor digitorum muscles.

Technique To a depth of about 0.3 cun; perpendicular insertion.

LI-9 Upper Ridge

上廉 *Shang Lian*

Effect Moves *qi* along the channel, harmonizes the large intestine.

Indications Pain in the shoulder and foreleg, carpal joint pain, edemas, headache, hemiplegia. For excessive mental effort.

Localization 3 cun below LI-11, on the belly of the extensor digitorum muscle.

Technique To a depth of about 1 cun; perpendicular insertion.

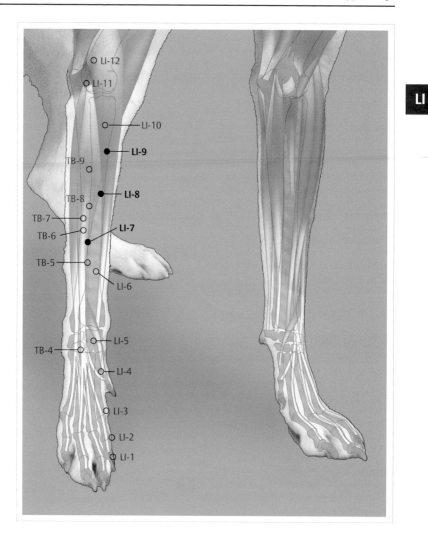

LI-10 Arm Three *Li*
手三里 *Shou San Li*

Effect Supplements and strengthens *qi*, resolves obstructions in the channel, harmonizes the stomach and intestine.

Indications Distal point for any problems in the path of the channel; for example, the elbow, carpal joint, shoulder, and side of the throat; inflammation in the throat, swollen lymph nodes; radial paralysis; abdominal pain; diarrhea; weakened immune system.

Localization 2 cun distal to LI-11, in an indentation at the edge of the extensor carpi radialis muscle.

Technique To a depth of about 1 cun; perpendicular insertion.

LI-11 Pool at the Bend
曲池 *Qu Chi*

He-sea point, earth point, supplementing point.

Effect Dispels wind and heat everywhere in the body, cools and regulates blood, regulates food (*gu*) *qi*, loosens phlegm, draws out dampness, relieves itching, supports the tendons and joints.

Indications Fever; chronic infectious disease; stimulates the immune system; urticaria; itching; dermatitis; pathologies of the endocrine system; localized problems in the elbow and shoulder; paralysis of the forehand; pharyngitis; pain or inflammation in the teeth, eyes, and nape; abdominal pain; spasms in the stomach and esophagus. Helps to release obsessive behaviors.

Localization In an indentation above the elbow, with the elbow slightly flexed, located in the crook of the arm in the middle between the lateral epicondyle of the humerus and the terminal tendon of the biceps muscle of the arm.

Technique To a depth of about 0.5 cun; perpendicular insertion.

LI-12 Elbow Bone-Hole
肘髎 *Zhou Liao*

Effect Moves *qi* along the channel, supports the elbow joint.

Indications Pain in the elbow and upper arm, radial paralysis. For inability to recognize possible actions.

Localization Laterally on the distal end of the humerus, on the dorsal edge of the lateral epicondyle.

Technique To a depth of about 0.5 cun; perpendicular insertion.

 Branches of the radial nerve lie underneath.

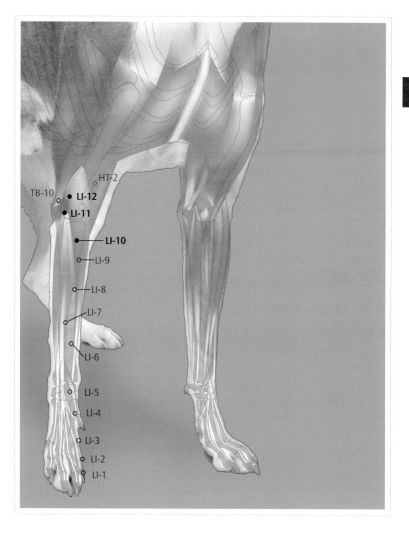

LI

LI-13 Arm Five *Li*
手五里 *Shou Wu Li*

Effect Regulates *qi*, transforms phlegm, draws out dampness, relieves coughing, moves *qi* along the channel.

Indications Pain in the shoulder, elbow, and upper arm; radial paralysis; lymphadenitis in the area of the neck; cough.

Localization Centrally in the lower third of the length of the humerus, between the belly of the brachial muscle and the lateral head of the triceps muscle of the arm, when standing straight about 2 cun above LI-11.

Technique To a depth of about 0.5 cun; perpendicular insertion.

LI-14 Upper Arm
臂臑 *Bi Nao*

Intersection point with the small intestine and bladder channels.

Effect Regulates *qi*, loosens phlegm, supports the eyes, moves *qi* along the channel.

Indications Pain in the shoulder and upper arm, atrophy of the upper arm muscles, goiter, visual disturbances.

Localization Lateral on the upper arm, at the beginning of the deltoid tuberosity.

Technique To a depth of about 0.5 cun; perpendicular insertion.

LI-15 Shoulder Bone
肩髃 *Jian Yu*

Intersection point with the *yang qiao mai* (*yang* springing vessel).

Effect Relaxes the tendons, promotes the flow of *qi* in the channel, dispels wind-damp, supports the shoulder, regulates *qi* and blood, loosens phlegm.

Indications Problems in the shoulder area, osteochondritis dissecans, diagnostic and therapeutic point for problems in the shoulder joint, atrophy or paralysis of the foreleg, hemiplegia, generalized exanthems.

Localization At the height of the shoulder joint, craniodistal to the acromion, on the front edge of the acromial head of the deltoid muscle.

Technique To a depth of about 0.3 cun; perpendicular insertion.

LI

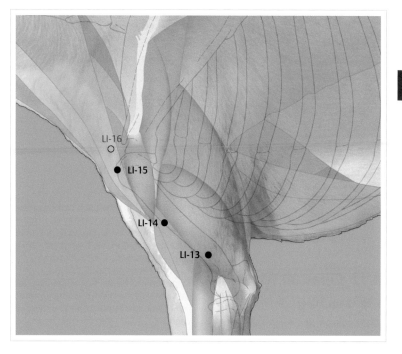

LI-16 Huge Bone
巨骨 *Ju Gu*

Intersection point with the *yang qiao mai* (*yang* springing vessel).

Effect Promotes the flow of *qi* in the channel, supports the shoulder, regulates *qi* and blood, loosens phlegm, stimulates the descent of lung *qi,* opens up the thorax.

Indications Pain in the shoulder, diagnostic and therapeutic point for problems in the shoulder joint, osteochondritis dissecans, toothache in the upper jaw, gingivitis.

Localization Lateral directly above the shoulder joint, directly above LI-15.

Technique To a depth of about 0.3 cun; perpendicular insertion.

LI-17 Celestial Tripod
天鼎 *Tian Ding*

Effect Supports the throat and voice.

Indications Pain in the shoulder, tonsillitis, laryngopharyngitis, inspiratory stridor, loss of voice. Supports transformation and connects upward.

Localization On the side of the neck about 1 cun below LI-18, following the neck line dorsal to the jugular groove at the level of the fifth cervical vertebra.

Technique To a depth of about 0.5 cun; perpendicular insertion.

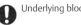 Underlying blood vessels.

LI-18 Protuberance Assistant
扶突 *Fu Tu*

Effect Supports the neck and voice, relieves coughing.

Indications Laryngopharyngitis, tracheo-bronchitis, difficulty swallowing, irritation of the throat with changed voice. For attachment to the past, suppressed expression of emotions.

Localization On the side of the neck dorsal to the jugular groove, where an imaginary extension of the lower jaw meets its edge.

Technique To a depth of about 0.5 cun; perpendicular insertion.

 Underlying blood vessels.

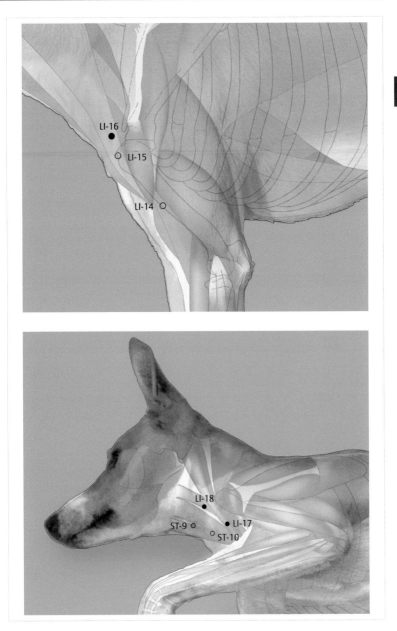

LI

LI-19 Grain Bone-Hole

禾髎 *He Liao*

Effect Eliminates wind, opens the nose.

LI

Indications Acute rhinitis, swollen nasal mucosa, bleeding, facial nerve paresis, trigeminal neuralgia, epiglottic entrapment, sinusitis.

Localization Lateroventral to the nostril and LI-20.

Technique To a depth of about 0.3 cun; oblique insertion in a rostral direction.

LI-20 Welcome Fragrance

迎香 *Ying Xiang*

Intersection point with the stomach channel.

Effect Dispels wind-heat, opens the nose and sinuses.

Indications Rhinitis, sinusitis, fever, facial nerve paresis, epistaxis, problems of the nasolacrimal duct, allergic bronchitis, and rhinitis. Release point. Strengthens instincts.

Localization In the middle of the lateral aspect nostril, on the border between nose and flew where the nostrils are widest.

Technique To a depth of about 0.3 cun; perpendicular insertion.

LI

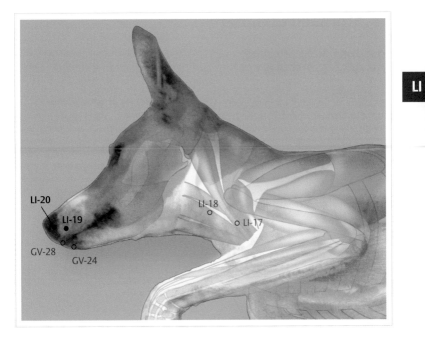

13 Stomach Channel

Foot *Yang Ming* (*Zu Yang Ming Wei* 足阳明胃脉)

The stomach channel starts at LI-2, runs from there to the inner canthus, meets up with the bladder channel at BL-1, and ascends along the eye sockets to ST-1 in the center of the edge of the lower eyelid. Then it meets up with the governing vessel (*du mai*), runs around the lips, continues laterally across the cheeks to ST-5 and ST-6, rises in front of the ear, rises further into the temporal area, and links up with GV-24.

At ST-5, a branch splits off and runs along the sternocleidomastoid muscle down the neck to enter the body at ST-12. It continues on to GV-14, then descends through the diaphragm, penetrates into the stomach, and connects with the spleen.

Another branch runs superficially from ST-12 lateral to the midline in a distal direction to ST-30 in the inguinal area.

Another branch starts at the pyloric opening of the stomach and meets with ST-30, then continues in a dorsal direction to ST-31 on the dorsolateral thigh below the iliac fossa, and then along the thigh in a distal direction to its final destination on the lateral side of the nail fold of the second hind toe.

The next branch splits off at ST-36 and ends in the foot.

A further branch splits off at ST-42 and ends on the lateral side of the third toe of the hind foot, to connect there with SP-1.

ST

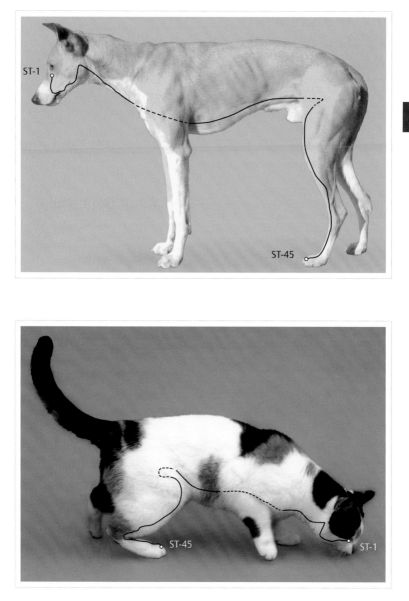

ST-1 Tear Container
承泣 Cheng Qi

Intersection point with the *yang* springing vessel (*yang qiao mai*) and controlling vessel (*ren mai*), local point.

Effect Draws wind and heat out of the eye, stops the flow of tears.

Indications Eye disorders, including chronic ones; sinusitis; rhinitis: facial nerve paralysis. Allows for the recognition and processing of past traumas.

Localization Centrally on the lower eyelid, on the conjunctival side between the ventral edge of the socket and the eyeball.

Technique To a depth of about 1 cun; perpendicular insertion below the eyeball along the socket, without injuring the eye.

 Do not needle in restless animals. Danger of injury.

ST-2 Four Whites
四白 Si Bai

Effect Draws wind and heat out of the eye.

Indications Eye disorders, facial nerve paresis, trigeminal neuralgia, sinusitis.

Localization On the infraorbital foramen, rostroventral to ST-1; the infraorbital nerve is located in the depth below.

Technique To a depth of about 0.5 cun; perpendicular insertion.

 Due to the risk of injuring the infraorbital nerve, do not stimulate the needle.

ST-3 Giant Bone-Hole
巨髎 Ju Liao

Intersection point with the *yang* springing vessel (*yang qiao mai*).

Effect Eliminates wind and swellings, moves *qi* along the channel.

Indications Facial nerve paresis, swollen flews, toothache, rhinitis, swelling in the knee.

Localization 1 cun below ST-2, in the flew above the third premolar.

Technique To a depth of about 0.3 cun; tangential insertion.

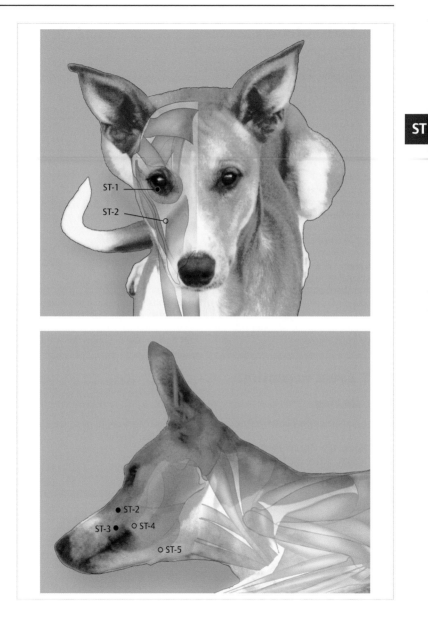

ST

ST-4 Earth Granary
地仓 *Di Cang*

Intersection point with the large intestine channel, the *yang* springing vessel (*yang qiao mai*), and the controlling vessel (*ren mai*).

Effect Draws external wind out of the face, calms muscles and tendons in the face, resolves obstructions in the channel.

Indications Facial nerve paralysis, trigeminal neuralgia, lockjaw, tetanus spasms, excessive salivation, eczema in the folds of the flews, eyelid spasms. Facilitates the appropriate communication and processing of problems. Calming point.

Localization A short distance behind the mucocutaneous transition in the lateral corner of the mouth, below the center of the pupil.

Technique To a depth of about 0.5 cun; perpendicular insertion.

ST-5 Great Reception
大迎 *Da Ying*

Effect Eliminates wind and swellings.

Indications Facial nerve paresis, trigeminal neuralgia, eyelid spasms, lockjaw, tetanus spasms, parotitis, swellings, toothache

in the lower jaw. Treats the psychological cause of lockjaw with determination to not accept any outside help.

Localization Lateral on the lower jaw in the facial vascular notch.

Technique To a depth of about 0.5 cun; perpendicular insertion.

 Underlying artery.

ST-6 Cheek Carriage
颊车 *Jia Che*

Effect Scatters wind, moves *qi* along the channel, moistens the larynx, supports the jaws and teeth.

Indications Facial nerve paralysis, lockjaw, toothache, masseter spasms, tetanus spasms, parotitis, salivary gland stones, stiff neck. Often in connection with rage, calms.

Localization In a depression in the masseter, just rostral to the jaw angle.

Technique To a depth of about 0.5 cun; perpendicular insertion.

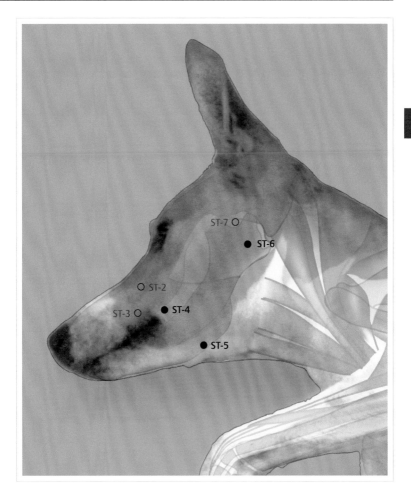

ST

ST-7 Below the Joint
下关 *Xia Guan*

Intersection point with the gallbladder channel.

Effect Moves *qi* along the channel, supports the jaws, ears, and teeth.

Indications Problems with the temporomandibular joint, temporomandibular joint arthrosis, facial nerve paresis, lockjaw, trigeminal neuralgia, otitis media with anger about inadequate care.

Localization Directly below the posterior part of the cheekbone in the mandibular notch.

Technique To a depth of about 0.3 cun; perpendicular insertion.

 Do not needle in a ventral direction; risk of inserting into the temporomandibular joint.

ST-8 Head Corner
头维 *Tou Wei*

Intersection point with the gallbladder channel and the *yang* linking vessel (*yang wei mai*).

Effect Eliminates wind-heat and obstructions of the channel, supports the eyes.

Indications Eye disorders, trigeminal neuralgia, facial nerve paresis.

Localization In the center of the temporal muscle on the line between the lateral canthus and the base of the ear.

Technique To a depth of about 0.2 cun; perpendicular insertion.

ST-9 Man's Prognosis
人迎 *Ren Ying*

Intersection point with the gallbladder channel, a point of the sea of *qi*.

Effect Regulates *qi* and blood, lowers rebellious *qi*, supports the throat and pharynx, moves *qi* along the channel, test point for the state of *yang, promotes openness to one's own needs and the needs of others.*

Indications Asthma, dyspnea, laryngitis, struma, hypertonicity. For refusing to eat (eating disorders), sexual dysfunctions, poisoning, heat stroke.

Localization Medial to the sternocleidomastoid muscle and the jugular vein, on the lower edge of the upper third of the length of the throat, below the thyroid cartilage.

Technique To a depth of about 0.5 cun; perpendicular insertion.

 Jugular vein.

ST

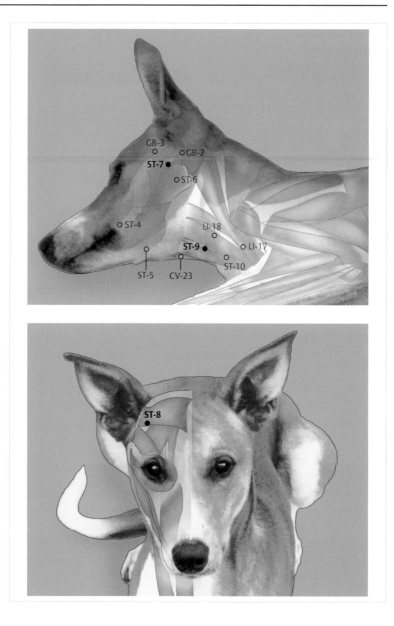

ST

ST-10 Water Prominence

水突 *Shui Tu*

Effect Lowers lung *qi*, supports the throat and pharynx.

Indications Angina, tonsillar abscess, cough, stiff neck, struma. Helpful in processing psychological problems that have started to shift.

Localization Medial to the sternocleidomastoid muscle and the jugular vein, in the middle of the length of the throat.

Technique To a depth of about 0.5 cun; perpendicular insertion.

 Jugular vein.

ST-11 *Qi* Abode

人迎 *Qi She*

Effect Lowers lung *qi*, supports the throat and pharynx.

Indications Chronic recurrent angina, cough, stiff neck, swollen lymph nodes of the neck.

Localization Lateral to the manubrium, at the base of the sternocleidomastoid muscle.

Technique To a depth of about 0.5 cun; perpendicular insertion.

ST-12 Empty Basin

缺盆 *Que Pen*

Intersection point with the large intestine, small intestine, triple burner, and gallbladder channels.

Effect Clears heat from the thorax and lowers rebellious lung *qi*, moves *qi* along the channel.

Indications Asthma, dyspnea, hypertonicity, intercostal neuralgia, problems with bringing the forelegs forward, pleuritis, angina, pharyngitis, ulcers in the stomach and small intestines. For identity crisis due to a change in living conditions and tasks.

Localization Lateral to the manubrium in the extension of the line of the mammary glands, in the jugular fossa.

Technique To a depth of about 0.5 cun; perpendicular insertion.

The points ST-13 to ST-27 lie on the mammillary line. If one of these points lies under a teat, needle it in front of or behind it. Do not needle in lactating teats.

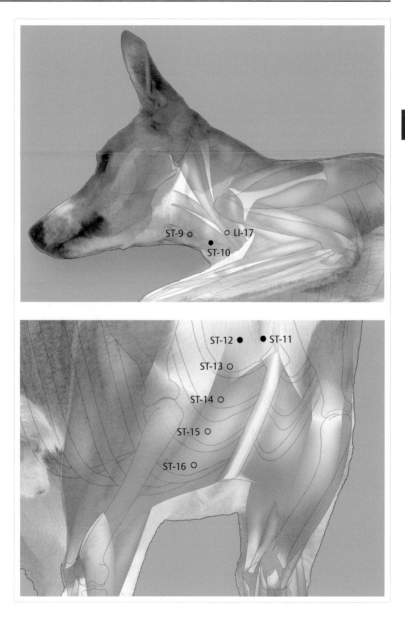

ST

ST-13 *Qi* Door
气户 *Qi Hu*

Effect   Lowers rebellious *qi* and opens up the thorax.

Indications   Dyspnea, cough, hypertonicity, heart problems, ulcers in the stomach and small intestine. Improves the ability to receive and express compassion.

Localization   Lateral to the sternum, caudal to the jugular fossa at the height of the first rib, 4 cun lateral to the midline on a line with the teats.

Technique   To a depth of about 0.5 cun; perpendicular insertion.

ST-14 Storeroom
库房 *Ku Fang*

Effect   Lowers rebellious *qi* and opens up the thorax.

Indications   Pain in the lateral thorax wall, cough with sputum, dyspnea, mastitis of the thoracic teat. Nourishes a deep need for affection.

Localization   In the first intercostal space, 4 cun lateral to the midline on a line with the teats.

Technique   To a depth of about 0.2 cun; perpendicular insertion.

 Risk of pneumothorax.

ST-15 Roof
屋翳 *Wu Yi*

Effect   Lowers rebellious *qi* and opens up the thorax, relieves itching of the skin, moves *qi* along the channel.

Indications   Pain in the lateral thorax wall, cough with sputum, dyspnea, mastitis of the thoracic teat, swollen teats. Provides emotional independence.

Localization   In the second intercostal space, 4 cun lateral to the midline on a line with the teats.

Technique   To a depth of about 0.2 cun; perpendicular insertion.

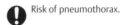 Risk of pneumothorax.

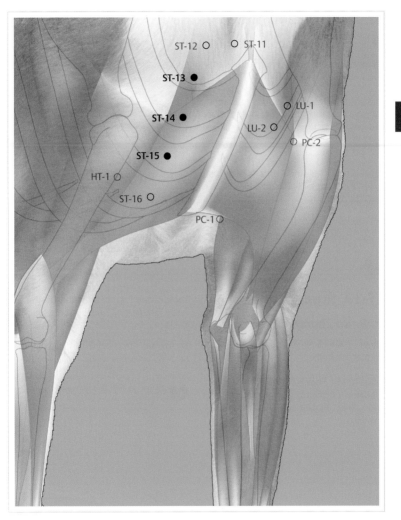

ST

ST

ST-16 Breast Window

膺窗 *Ying Chuang*

Effect Calms coughing and panting, supports the mammae.

Indications Regional rib pain, cough, shortness of breath, sleep disorders, fever and chills, watery diarrhea, mammary abscess. Opens one up emotionally to the outside, to giving.

Localization In the third intercostal space, 4 cun lateral to the midline on a line with the teats.

Technique To a depth of about 0.2 cun; perpendicular insertion.

 Risk of pneumothorax.

ST-17 Breast Center

乳中 *Ru Zhong*

Effect Calms coughing and panting, supports the mammae.

Indications Regional rib pain, cough, shortness of breath, sleep disorders, fever and chills, watery diarrhea, mammary abscess.

Localization In the fourth intercostal space, 4 cun lateral to the midline on a line with the teats.

Technique To a depth of about 0.2 cun; perpendicular insertion.

 Risk of pneumothorax.

ST-18 Breast Root

乳根 *Ru Gen*

Effect Calms coughing and panting, supports the mammae, eliminates swelling.

Indications Regional rib pain, cough, shortness of breath, blockage in the area of the diaphragm, mastitis of the thoracic teats. Promotes the ability to give.

Localization In the fifth intercostal space, 4 cun lateral to the midline on a line with the teats.

Technique To a depth of about 0.2 cun; perpendicular insertion.

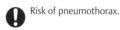 Risk of pneumothorax.

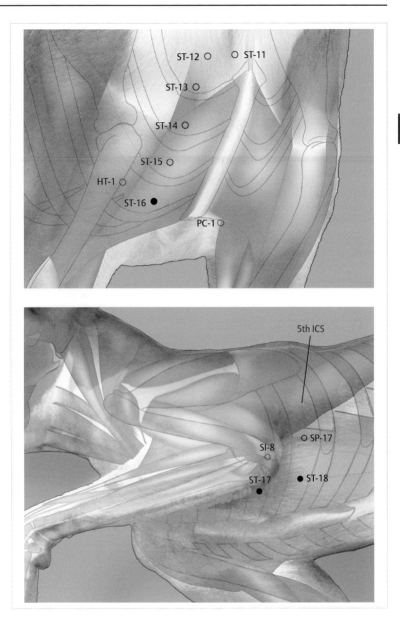

ST-12 ○   ○ ST-11

ST-13 ○

ST-14 ○

ST-15 ○

HT-1 ○

ST-16 ●

PC-1 ○

5th ICS

○ SP-17

SI-8 ○

ST-17 ●   ● ST-18

ST-19 Not Contained

不容 *Bu Rong*

Effect Harmonizes the middle burner, lowers rebellious *qi*, lowers lung *qi*, relieves panting.

Indications Regional rib pain, cough, shortness of breath, blockage in the area of the diaphragm, nausea, abdominal pain, mastitis of the thoracic teats. Helps in concluding thoughts.

Localization In the ninth intercostal space, 4 cun lateral to the midline on a line with the teats.

Technique To a depth of about 0.2 cun; perpendicular insertion.

❗ Risk of pneumothorax.

ST-20 Assuming Fullness

承满 *Cheng Man*

Effect Harmonizes the middle burner, lowers rebellious lung and stomach *qi*.

Indications Regional rib pain, abdominal pain and spasms, tension in the abdominal wall, mastitis of the thoracic teats. Fills inner emptiness and the need for affection.

Localization In the tenth intercostal space, 4 cun lateral to the midline on a line with the teats.

Technique To a depth of about 0.2 cun; perpendicular insertion.

❗ Risk of pneumothorax.

ST-21 Beam Gate

梁门 *Liang Men*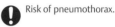

Effect Regulates the stomach and suppresses rebellious *qi*, harmonizes the middle burner, and resolves stagnation.

Indications Abdominal pain, abdominal ulcers, lack of appetite, all forms of digestive disorders, regional rib pain, mastitis in regional mammary complexes. Brings movement to digestive processes that have gotten stuck at every level.

Localization In the 11th intercostal space, 4 cun lateral to the midline on a line with the teats.

Technique To a depth of about 0.2 cun; tangential insertion.

 Puncture of the abdominal cavity.

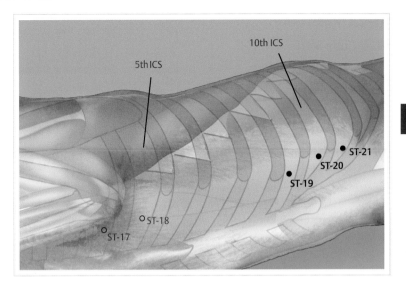

ST-22 Pass Gate
关门 *Guan Men*

Effect Regulates *qi* and moves it along the channel, supports the intestines and urination.

Indications All forms of digestive disorders, regional rib pain, mastitis in regional teats, urinary incontinence. Helps at the psychological level with processing change and releasing the old.

Localization In the 12th intercostal space, 4 cun lateral to the midline on a line with the teats.

Technique To a depth of about 0.2 cun; tangential insertion.

 Puncture of the abdominal cavity.

ST-23 Supreme Unity
太一 *Tai Yi*

Effect Harmonizes the middle burner, transforms phlegm, calms the spirit.

Indications Abdominal pain and ulcers, digestive disorders, vomiting, mastitis in regional mammary complexes. Facilitates a view of everything and the integration thereof.

Localization Below the 13th rib, 4 cun lateral to the midline on a line with the teats.

Technique To a depth of about 0.2 cun; tangential insertion.

 Puncture of the abdominal cavity.

ST-24 Slippery Flesh Gate
滑肉门 *Hua Rou Men*

Effect Harmonizes the stomach, transforms phlegm, suppresses rebellious stomach *qi*, calms the spirit.

Indications Pain and functional disorders in the stomach and small intestine, vomiting, mastitis in regional mammary complexes. Provides nourishment also at the emotional level.

Localization On the mammary line halfway between ST-23 and ST-25 or the navel.

Technique To a depth of about 0.2 cun; tangential insertion.

 Puncture of the abdominal cavity.

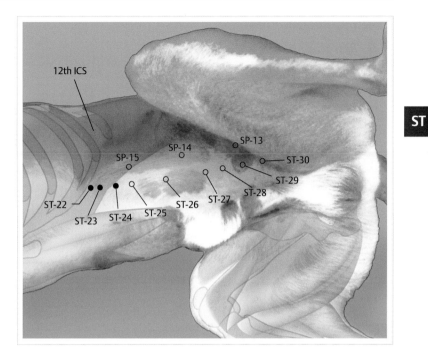

ST

ST-25 Celestial Pivot

天枢 *Tian Shu*

Mu-alarm point of the large intestine.

Effect   Normalizes the transport function of the large intestine, regulates the spleen and stomach, eliminates damp-heat, regulates *qi* and blood, removes stagnation.

Indications   Acute and chronic gastrointestinal disorders, lack of appetite, vomiting, abdominal masses, mastitis, ascites. Stabilizes mentally and emotionally, as well as at the level of the *shen*. For inner turmoil and mood swings.

Localization   2 cun lateral to the center of the navel.

Technique   To a depth of about 0.2 cun; tangential insertion.

 Puncture of the abdominal cavity.

ST-26 Outer Mound

外陵 *Wai Ling*

Effect   Regulates *qi* and moves it along the channel.

Indications   Acute and chronic gastrointestinal disorders, abdominal pain, colic, ovarian cysts, mastitis. When not becoming pregnant and against rejecting the mother's role.

Localization   On the mammary line, halfway between ST-25 and ST-27.

Technique   To a depth of about 0.2 cun; tangential insertion.

 Puncture of the abdominal cavity.

ST-27 Great Gigantic

大巨 *Da Ju*

Effect   Regulates *qi*, supports the kidneys and essence, promotes urination.

Indications   Functional disorders of the large intestine and urogenital tract, diarrhea, mastitis of the posterior mammary complexes, edemas, and for depressions in this context.

Localization   On the mammary line, where it meets the vertical line to the coxal tuber.

Technique   To a depth of about 0.2 cun; tangential insertion.

 Puncture of the abdominal cavity.

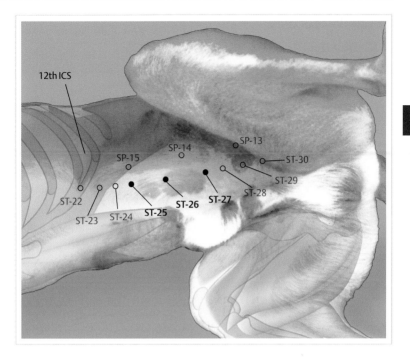

ST-28 Waterway

水道 *Shui Dao*

Effect Regulates the lower burner, removes stagnation, supports the bladder and uterus.

Indications Functional disorders of the urogenital tract, edemas, cystitis, orchitis, mastitis in the inguinal teat complex, gastritis, urinary retention, and obsessive movements of turning in circles.

Localization On the mammary line, in the first third of the distance between ST-27 and ST-30.

Technique To a depth of about 0.2 cun; tangential insertion.

 Puncture of the abdominal cavity.

ST-29 Return

归来 *Gui Lai*

Effect Warms the lower burner, supports the genitals.

Indications Cryptorchism, hernias, impotence, functional disorders of the urogenital tract, mastitis in the inguinal teats. Regulates all cyclical constructive and deconstructive processes, pulls back prolapses.

Localization On the mammary line, in the second third of the distance between ST-27 and ST-30.

Technique To a depth of about 0.2 cun; tangential insertion.

ST-30 *Qi* Thoroughfare

气冲 *Qi Chong*

Intersection point with the thoroughfare vessel (*chong mai*), a point of the sea of grain, connects the superficial course of the channel to the deeper course.

Effect Regulates *qi* in the lower burner and moves into the hind legs, strengthens essence, regulates stomach *qi* and the blood.

Indications Functional disorders of the sexual organs, obstetric complications, mastitis in the inguinal teats, lack of appetite, inefficient feed conversion, meteorism. Restores zest for life, moves stagnation.

Localization In front of the pectineal line of the pubis, lateral to the midline, cranial to the inguinal canal.

Technique To a depth of about 0.3 cun; tangential insertion.

ST

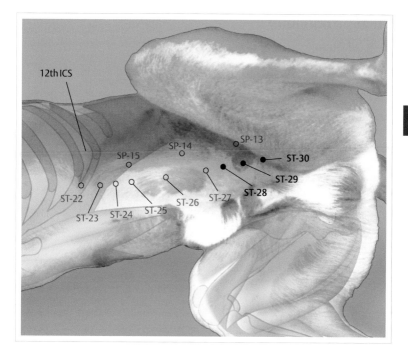

ST

ST-31 Thigh Joint
髀关 *Bi Guan*

Effect   Expels wind-damp, moves *qi* and blood along the channel and out of the abdominal space into the hind legs.

Indications   Paresis of the hind legs, hip joint dysplasia, lumbago, knee problems, lymph congestion in the inguinal area.

Localization   On the cranial edge of the thigh approximately at the end of the upper third of the distance between the upper edge of the patella and the coxal tuber, between the lateral edge of the sartorius muscle and tensor muscles of fasciae latae.

Technique   To a depth of about 0.5 cun; perpendicular insertion.

ST-32 Crouching Rabbit
伏兔 *Fu Tu*

Effect   Expels wind-damp, moves *qi* along the channel.

Indications   Pareses of the hind legs, muscle atrophy, hip joint dysplasia, lumbago, knee problems, urticaria. With Ren-15,

ST-25, ST-32, and ST-41 bilaterally (seven dragon points), this is the classical treatment for obsessions and possessiveness.

Localization   On the cranial edge of the thigh approximately on the border of the lower quarter of the distance between the upper edge of the patella and the coxal tuber, on the muscle–tendon border of the rectus femoris muscle.

Technique   To a depth of about 0.5 cun; perpendicular insertion.

ST-33 *Yin* Market
阴市 *Yin Shi*

Effect   Expels wind-damp, moves *qi* along the channel.

Indications   Pareses and spasms in the hind legs, muscle atrophy, lumbago, knee joint problems, abdominal pain, ascites, pancreas problems. For movement in cases of strong lethargy.

Localization   Approximately 2 cun above the patella between the rectus femoris and vastus lateralis muscles.

Technique   To a depth of about 0.5 cun; perpendicular insertion.

ST

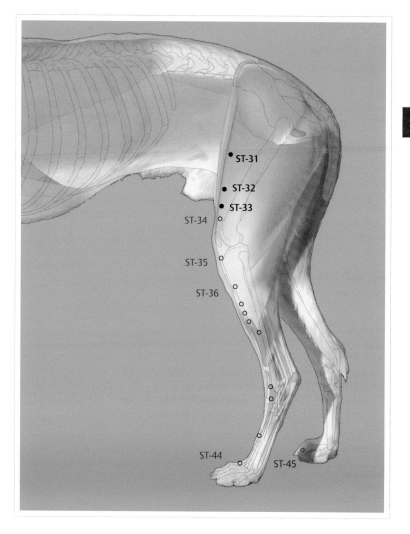

ST-31

ST-32

ST-33

ST-34

ST-35

ST-36

ST-44   ST-45

ST-34 Beam Hill

梁丘 *Liang Qiu*

Xi-cleft point.

Effect Moves *qi* along the channel, harmonizes the stomach, eases acute conditions.

Indications Pareses and spasms in the hind legs, muscle atrophy, lumbago, knee joint problems, abdominal pain, mastitis. Activates earth energies to pull depression out of the hole or to ground mania.

Localization Approximately 1 cun above the patella between the rectus femoris and vastus lateralis muscles.

Technique To a depth of about 0.3 cun; perpendicular insertion.

ST-35 Calf's Nose

犊鼻 *Du Bi*

In connection with the corresponding medial extra point, it is also called lateral knee eye or *xi yan*.

Effect Moves *qi* along the channel; local point for the knee; draws out dampness, swelling, and cold.

Indications Knee pain; gonarthrosis, especially on the front of the knee or deep inside the joint. Transforms rigidity into adaptability.

Localization In the depression below the patella, lateral to the patellar ligament.

Technique To a depth of about 0.3 cun; perpendicular or slightly oblique insertion in a distal direction.

ST-36 Leg Three *Li*

足三里 *Zu San Li*

He-sea point, earth point, a point of the sea of grain.

Effect Normalizes the down-leading function of the stomach; supports the spleen's functions of transformation and transport; expels cold; lifts up *yang*; supplements *qi*; nourishes *yuan qi*, blood, and *yin*; calms the spirit; moves *qi* along the channel.

Indications All gastrointestinal problems, stomach or biliary colic, impaired digestion, knee problems, tibial and fibular paralysis, immunodeficiency, tendency to infection, fever, anorexia, lethargy, asthma. Strengthens earth energy through supplementation in cases of deficiency and exhaustion. Connects to the here and now.

Localization 3 cun distal to ST-35, laterally at the height of the distal end of the tibial tuberosity, in a depression roughly in the center of the tibialis cranialis muscle.

Technique To a depth of about 1 cun; perpendicular insertion.

ST

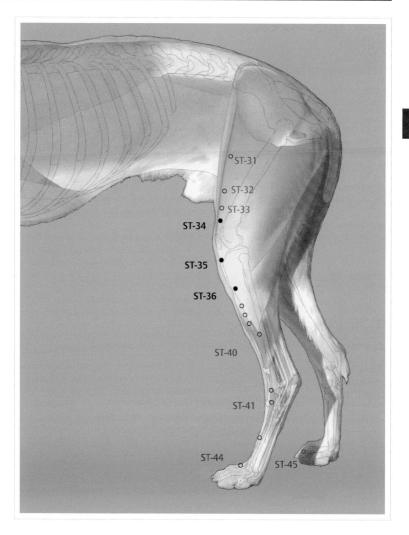

ST-31
ST-32
ST-33
ST-34
ST-35
ST-36
ST-40
ST-41
ST-44   ST-45

ST

ST-37 Upper Great Hollow

上巨虛 *Shang Ju Xu*

A point of the sea of blood, lower *he*-sea point of the large intestine.

Effect Regulates the spleen, intestines, and stomach; clears damp-heat; removes food stagnation; moves *qi* along the channel; pain in the knee and ankle.

Indications Digestive disorders, stomach cramps, obstipation, meteorism, diarrhea.

Localization Below the knee, 3 cun underneath ST-36, centered in the tibialis cranialis muscle.

Technique To a depth of about 1 cun; perpendicular insertion.

ST-38 Ribbon Opening

条口 *Tiao Kou*

Effect Moves *qi* along the channel, draws out wind-damp, supports the shoulder region.

Indications Digestive disorders, stomach cramps, obstipation, meteorism, diarrhea, ipsilateral shoulder pain, pain in the knee.

Localization On the lower leg on the tibialis cranialis muscle, halfway along the distance between the lower edge of the patella and the lateral malleolus.

Technique To a depth of about 1 cun; perpendicular insertion.

ST-39 Lower Great Hollow

下巨虛 *Xia Ju Xu*

A point of the sea of blood, lower *he*-sea point of the small intestine channel.

Effect Harmonizes the intestines, moves the *qi* of the small intestine, clears wind and damp-heat, moves *qi* along the channel, for states of deficiency in the lower burner.

Indications Digestive disorders, gastrointestinal colic, colitis, enteritis, meteorism, diarrhea, shoulder pain, muscle atrophy in the hind legs.

Localization On the lateral posterior lower leg on the tibialis cranialis muscle, 1 cun distal to ST-38.

Technique To a depth of about 1 cun; perpendicular insertion.

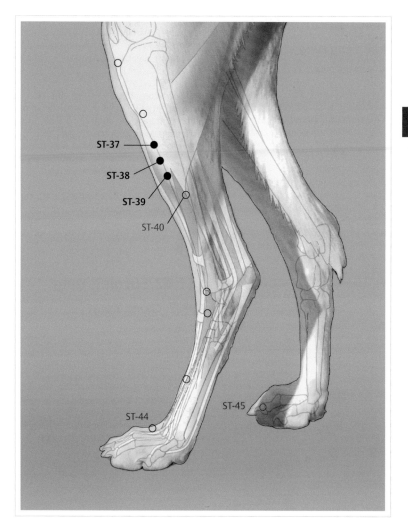

ST-37
ST-38
ST-39
ST-40
ST-44
ST-45

ST

ST-40 Bountiful Bulge
丰隆 *Feng Long*

Luo-network point.

Effect Transforms and resolves phlegm and dampness, clears heat (especially heat in the stomach), calms the spirit, opens up the chest, moves *qi* along the channel.

Indications Problems with phlegm in the respiratory tract, asthma, lumps everywhere, mental problems, pancreatic insufficiency, hepatopathy, epilepsy, swellings, pain and paralysis in the hind legs, phlegm in the body and below the skin, lipomas, goiter. Helps with feelings of inadequate care, which lead to attachment to the past or fixation on the future. In conjunction with SP-4, it opens the awareness of being provided for in the here and now.

Localization 8 cun proximal to the lateral malleolus, directly cranial to the fibula, 1 cun lateral to ST-38, between the tibialis cranialis and the long extensor muscles of the toes.

Technique To a depth of about 1 cun; perpendicular insertion.

ST-41 Ravine Divide
解溪 *Jie Xi*

Jing-river point, fire point, supplementing point.

Effect Resolves obstructions from the channel, eliminates wind, clears heat (especially stomach heat), clears the consciousness.

Indications Pain and swelling in the ankle, pain in the epigastrium, headache

and inflamed throat due to stomach heat, seizures, gastrointestinal flaccidity, tympanites. Breaks open obsessive behavior patterns. For mental confusion with signs of heat.

Localization Dorsal on the hind paw at the height of the heel, in the middle of the dorsal transverse ankle fold that forms during flexion, between the tendons of the long extensor muscles of the toes and the tibialis cranialis muscle, approximately at the level of the tip of the malleolus.

Technique To a depth of about 0.2 cun; perpendicular insertion.

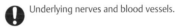 Underlying nerves and blood vessels.

ST-42 Surging *Yang*
冲阳 *Chong Yang*

Yuan-source point.

Effect Moves *qi* along the channel, clears heat from the channel, strengthens the stomach and spleen, calms the spirit.

Indications Pain and swelling in the ankle, paralyses, stomach problems, vomiting, facial nerve paresis, toothache. Helps with serious attention-seeking behavioral problems.

Localization Dorsal on the tarsal joint, distal to ST-41 below the trochlea of the talus, between the tendons of the long extensor muscles of the toes and tibialis cranialis muscle.

Technique To a depth of about 0.3 cun; perpendicular insertion.

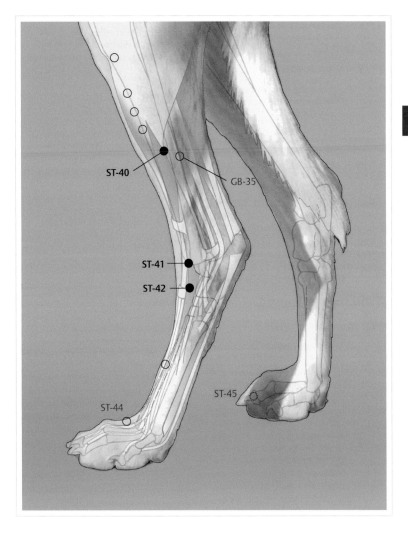

ST

ST

ST-43 Sunken Valley

陷谷 *Xian Gu*

Shu-stream point, wood point.

Effect Moves *qi* along the channel, expels wind-damp, harmonizes the stomach and spleen, removes swellings.

Indications Tendency to edemas, pain and swelling in the paw, abdominal pain, discharging and calming in fever (*yang ming* stage).

Localization Dorsal on the paw between the third and fourth metatarsal bones, approximately halfway up their length.

Technique To a depth of about 0.3 cun; perpendicular insertion.

ST-44 Inner Court

内庭 *Nei Ting*

Ying-brook point, water point.

Effect Clears heat from the channel and stomach, eliminates wind from the face; in "true heat and false cold": only the front or rear paws are cold, the rest of the body is warm; heat that is concentrated on the inside prevents *yang qi* from circulating freely into the extremities; pulse and tongue suggest cold; differential diagnosis; cold inversion, the entire extremity or the area below the knee/elbow is cold; spirit-calming.

Indications Painful swellings in the paw, toothache in the upper jaw, trigeminal neuralgia and facial nerve paralysis (in combination with LI-4), stomach problems due to heat, foul-smelling diarrhea, tonsillitis, mastitis. When fear due to weakness in earth floods the psyche. For phobias and withdrawal. Often observed in animal rescue cases.

Localization Dorsal on the paw, directly proximal to the edge of the thin skin between the third and fourth toes of the hind paw, in a depression laterodistal to the second metatarsophalangeal joint.

Technique To a depth of about 0.3 cun; perpendicular insertion.

ST-45 Severe Mouth

厉兑 *Li Dui*

Jing-well point, metal point, sedation point.

Effect Disperses heat from the stomach channel, regulates *qi*, resolves and removes food stagnation, calms the spirit.

Indications Localized problems, pain and swelling in the paw, distal point for knee problems, dry mouth, gingivitis, tonsillitis, facial nerve paresis, trigeminal neuralgia, swollen flews, gastrointestinal problems, gastrointestinal ulcers, fever, hepatopathies, ascites. For emotionally isolating behavior, loss of contact, egocentrism, indifference. Demands a treat for every step.

Localization Lateral to the third hind toe next to the base of the nail.

Technique To a depth of about 0.2 cun; oblique insertion toward proximal.

ST

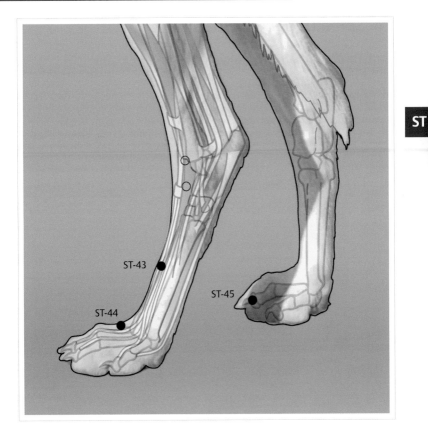

ST-43

ST-45

ST-44

14 Spleen/Pancreas Channel

Foot *Tai Yin (Zu Tai Yin Pi Mai* 足太阴脾脉)

The spleen channel begins medially on the second toe of the hind paw. Because dogs often lack this toe, it is under discussion whether points 1 to 3 are lost or whether they are located exactly medial to the second toe. The channel ascends along the medial hind leg, initially on the posterior edge of the tibia, crosses the liver channel 8 cun proximal to the medial malleolus, runs medially across the knee, and then runs anteromedially across the thigh up to the abdomen. From there, the channel enters the spleen and stomach. In the stomach area, it resurfaces and ascends lateral to the midline until it ends, after turning back in a caudal direction, in the sixth intercostal space in the axillary plane.

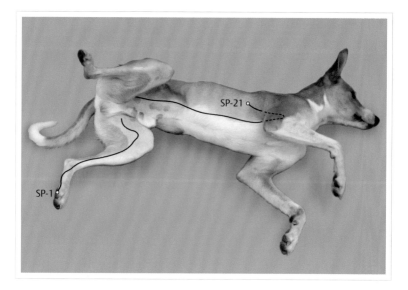

SP

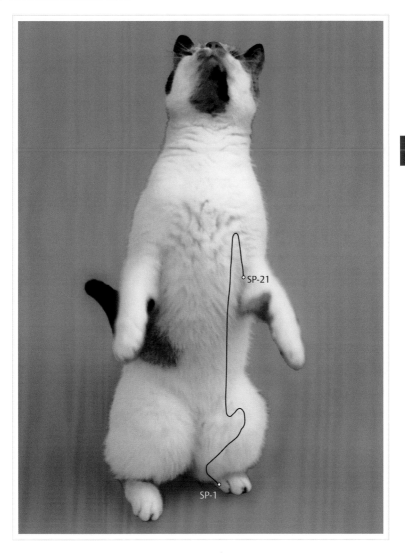

SP-1 *Yin* White
阴白 *Yin Bai*

Jing-well point, wood point.

Effect Strengthens the spleen, quickens the blood, stanches bleeding.

Indications Local point, generalized muscle disorders along the channel; in cases with chronic lack of appetite, chronic diarrhea, chronic hemorrhaging in the intestine and uterus. For loss of consciousness and weak concentration and memory. When rage prevents clear thinking and approachability.

Localization Varies in the literature between medial to the toe joint of the second toe of the hind paw between the distal and medial phalanges and, if present, in the medial claw fold of the first toe.

Technique To a depth of about 0.2 cun; deep perpendicular insertion.

SP-2 Great Metropolis
大都 *Da Du*

Ying-brook point, fire point, supplementing point.

Effect Supplementing point, eliminates heat and dampness, promotes digestion.

Indications Heat symptoms, febrile infections, local pain in the ankle, hot edemas.

Promotes inspiration and a warm heart in psychological issues.

Localization On the medial side of the second toe of the hind paw in the upper area of the proximal phalanx.

Technique To a depth of about 0.2 cun; perpendicular insertion.

SP-3 Supreme White
太白 *Tai Bai*

Shu-stream point, earth point, *yuan*-source point.

Effect Strengthens earth and the spleen and stomach, strengthens the spleen's functions of transformation and transport, and thereby dries dampness.

Indications All degenerative disorders of the body such as muscle atrophy, anemia, pareses of the hind legs, pancreatic insufficiency, diarrhea, debility. Clears the head and the thoughts.

Localization In dogs and cats, the first toe of the hind paw is either completely absent or only present in rudimentary form. We therefore find the point SP-3 caudomedially on the second metatarsal bone.

Technique To a depth of about 0.3 cun; oblique insertion upward from behind and below.

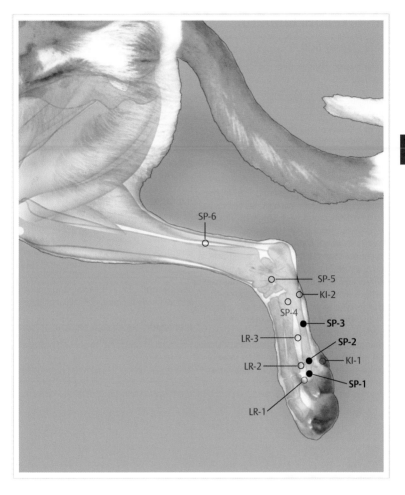

SP-4 Yellow Emperor

公孙 *Gong Sun*

Luo-network point, opener of the thoroughfare vessel (*chong mai*), and intersection point with the *yin* linking vessel (*yin wei mai*).

Effect Supplements the spleen and stomach, stanches bleeding, removes obstructions, regulates and eliminates dampness.

Indications Gastritis, digestive disorders, diarrhea, fertility problems, sphincter spasms, can facilitate parturition, retained placenta, testicular pain, problems with salivation, esophageal spasms, vocal cord spasms, heart pain, convulsant states, ankle problems. Helps with psychological programs caused by inadequate mothering. In conjunction with ST-40, it releases traumas in this context. SP-4 + SP-6 for analgesia.

Localization Medial in a depression that is distal and slightly plantar to the proximal end of the first metatarsal bone; if the first phalanx does not exist, then exactly medial to the base of the second metatarsal bone.

Technique To a depth of about 0.3 cun; oblique insertion upward from behind and below.

SP-5 *Shang* Hill

商丘 *Shang Qiu*

Sedation point, *jing*-river point, metal point.

Effect Strengthens the spleen and stomach, eliminates dampness.

Indications Gastrointestinal disorders, flatulence, meteorism, local point, soft tissue injuries in this area, weakness of the connective tissue, rectal prolapse. For insomnia due to large numbers of unprocessed ideas that cannot be implemented.

Localization In a depression below and behind the distal and medial tibial malleolus.

Technique To a depth of about 0.2 cun; perpendicular insertion.

SP

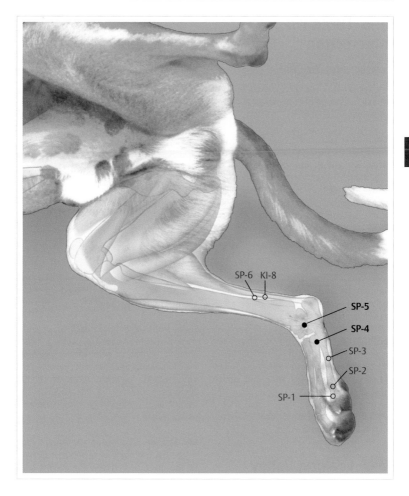

SP

SP-6 Three *Yin* Intersection
三阴交 *San Yin Jiao*

Meeting point of the three *yin* channels of the foot, master point of the lower abdomen and urogenital system.

Effect Normalizes the spleen's function of transformation and transport, transforms dampness and heat as well as phlegm and phlegm-heat, strengthens the control of *shen* via fluid metabolism, strengthens the harmonious flow of *gan qi*, calms the spirit, and strengthens the blood.

Indications Functional disorders of the urogenital system, dysentery, incontinence, weak contractions, triggers contractions, immunodeficiency, problems in the lower back. Helpful for *yin* depression with a feeling of heaviness due to excessive worrying.

Localization 3 cun directly above the center of the medial tibial malleolus, on the caudal edge of the tibia, on a line between the malleolus and SP-9, across from GB-39.

Technique To a depth of about 0.4 cun; perpendicular insertion.

SP-7 Leaking Valley
漏谷 *Lou Gu*

Effect Strengthens the spleen, eliminates dampness.

Indications Insufficient circulation or spasms in the hind legs, knee pain, maldigestion, meteorism. Helpful when emptiness in earth is unable to stabilize the memory and when it is impossible to implement learned skills.

Localization Central on the caudal edge of the tibia, halfway between the medial condyle and the medial malleolus.

Technique To a depth of about 0.5 cun; perpendicular insertion.

SP-8 Earth Winnower
地箕 *Di Ji*

Xi-cleft point.

Effect Removes obstructions from the channel, regulates *qi* and blood, regulates the uterus, relieves pain.

Indications Knee pain, lack of appetite, ascites, diarrhea, lumbago, sterility, oligospermia, abdominal pain, master point for functional urogenital disorders, uterine prolapse, uterine bleeding, incontinence. For compulsive striving for independence and immutable reaction patterns, extreme stubbornness.

Localization Central on the caudal edge of the tibia, at the end of the first quarter of the distance between the medial condyle and the medial malleolus.

Technique To a depth of about 0.5 cun; perpendicular insertion.

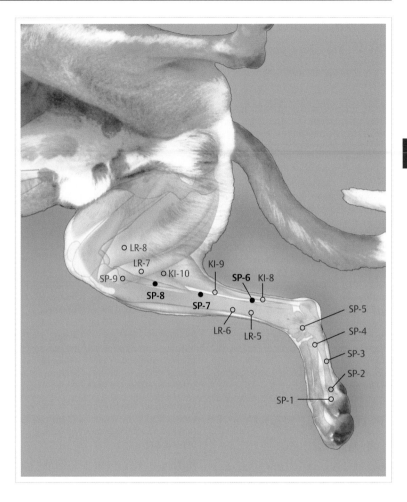

SP

SP-9 *Yin* Mound Spring

阴陵泉 *Yin Ling Quan*

He-sea point, water point, local point for the knee.

Effect Normalizes the spleen's functions of transformation and transport, eliminates dampness, transforms and draws out phlegm and phlegm-heat, especially in the lower burner.

Indications Gonarthrosis and arthritis, circulatory disorders in the hindquarters, abdominal pain with diarrhea, spasms, obstipation, disturbed urination, dysuria, ureteral colic, prostatitis, urogenital problems, ascites, all kinds of edemas, distal point for treating shoulder pain. Promotes openness to attention, in giving and receiving.

Localization On the lower edge of the medial condyle of the tibia, in a depression between the posterior edge of the tibia and the gastrocnemius muscle across from GB-34.

Technique To a depth of 1 cun; perpendicular insertion.

SP-10 Sea of Blood

血海 *Xue Hai*

Effect Resolves obstructions in the channel; calms the spirit; eliminates blood stasis, especially in the uterus; cools blood in cases of blood heat; nourishes the blood.

Indications Important point for stimulating the immune system, allergies, urticaria, bleeding, infectious diseases, estrus problems, improves circulation in the knee and hind legs. For insecurity and rejection of mating with spleen *qi* deficiency.

Localization With the knee bent, 2 cun above the craniomedial edge of the patella, on the belly of the cranial aspect of the sartorius muscle; on the cranial edge of the femur, on the tip of the vastus medialis muscle.

Technique To a depth of about 1 cun; perpendicular insertion.

SP-11 Winnower Gate

箕门 *Ji Men*

Effect Strengthens the function of the spleen, draws out dampness and heat.

Indications Improves circulation in the hind legs; paralysis of the hind legs, incontinence, pain and swelling in the inguinal area, urinary problems, abdominal pain with colic and/or diarrhea.

Localization Medial, central on the posterior edge of the femur between the sartorius and gracilis muscles above the femoral artery.

Technique To a depth of about 0.5 cun; insert perpendicularly **caudal** (!) to the femoral artery.

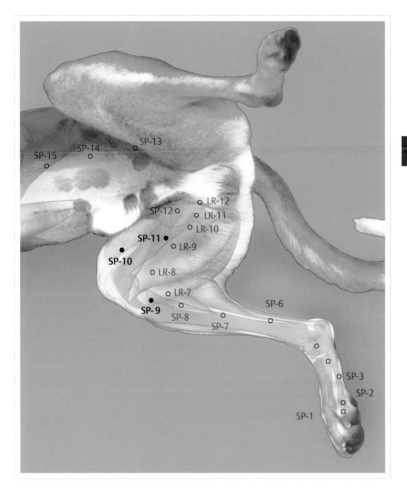

SP

SP

SP-12 Surging Gate
冲门 *Chong Men*

Connects the spleen and liver channels with the *yin* linking vessel (*yin wei mai*).

Effect Strengthens the function of the spleen, draws out dampness and heat.

Indications Pain and swelling in the inguinal area, hernias, problems in the kidneys or bladder and ureter, orchitis, intestinal spasms, endometriosis, postpartum bleeding, weak lactation. For self-pity and obsession due to spleen *qi* stagnation.

Localization In front of the pectineal line of the pubis in the groin cranial to the acetabulum.

Technique

 Because of the large blood vessels, do not needle.

SP-13 Bowel Abode
府舍 *Fu She*

Connects the spleen and liver channels with the *yin* linking vessel (*yin wei mai*).

Effect Moves *qi* along the channel.

Indications Hernias, piercing pain in the lower abdomen, digestive disorders, obstipation, kidney problems. For loss of the center and centralization, constant attention-seeking.

Localization 1 cun cranial to SP-12 and 4 cun lateral to the midline, at the height of CV-3, on the inner side of the beginning of the lateral umbilical fold.

Technique To a depth of about 0.5 cun; perpendicular insertion.

SP-14 Abdominal Bind
腹结 *Fu Jie*

Effect Regulates *qi*, lowers it, supports the lower burner.

Indications Abdominal pain in the umbilical area, acute diarrhea, respiratory problems with cough, excessive sweating, hernias, kidney problems. For frustration and dammed up rage in the abdomen.

Localization In the middle of a line from SP-13 to SP-15, on the inside of the lateral fold about 4 cun lateral to the midline and on the lateral edge of the rectus abdominis muscle.

Technique To a depth of about 0.5 cun; perpendicular insertion.

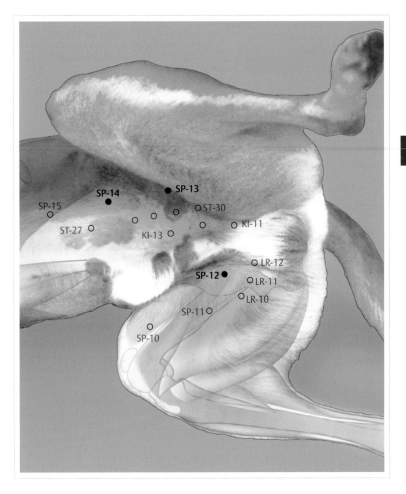

SP-15 Great Horizontal

大横 *Da Heng*

Connects to the *yin* linking vessel (*yin wei mai*).

Effect Strengthens the spleen and extremities, eliminates dampness, regulates the flow of *qi*, promotes the function of the large intestine.

Indications Strong diarrhea with meteorism, atonic obstipation, hernias, epileptiform attacks, excessive sweating. For emotional instability and senseless mood swings.

Localization Lateral to the navel, an additional 2 cun lateral to ST-25 on the lateral edge of the rectus abdominis muscle, where the lateral fold ends.

Technique To a depth of about 0.5 cun; perpendicular insertion.

SP-16 Abdominal Lament

腹哀 *Fu Ai*

Connects to the *yin* linking vessel (*yin wei mai*).

Effect Regulates the intestines.

Indications Digestive problems in the stomach, pancreatic insufficiency, colitis, abdominal pain. For stuck grief after miscarriage, also for depression during pregnancy.

Localization On the same level as SP-15 behind the caudal edge of the 12th rib.

Technique To a depth of about 0.3 cun; slightly oblique insertion forward.

SP-17 Food Hole

食窦 *Shi Dou*

Effect Eliminates retention of food and fluids.

Indications Thorax pain and feeling of fullness in the area of the diaphragm, dyspnea, mastitis. Helpful for processing an excessive abundance of information.

Localization In the fifth intercostal space on an imaginary contour line 2 cun below the height of the shoulder joint.

Technique To a depth of about 0.3 cun; oblique insertion forward.

 Risk of pneumothorax.

SP

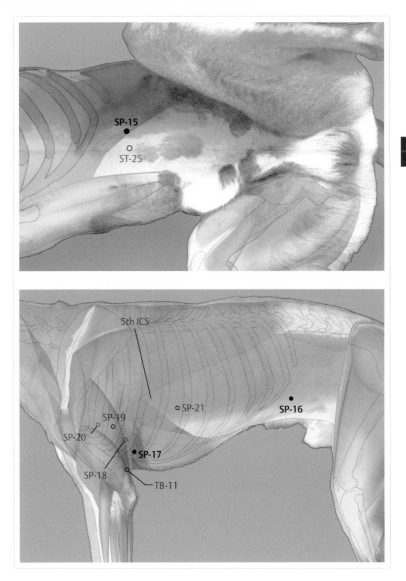

SP-18 Celestial Ravine

天溪 *Tian Xi*

Effect Local effect on the *qi* in the channel.

Indications Thorax pain, cough, dyspnea, mastitis if the anterior mammary complexes are affected, weakened lactation.

Localization In the fourth intercostal space on an imaginary contour line 1.5 cun below the height of the shoulder joint in the armpit.

Technique

 Do not needle: risk of pneumothorax.

SP-19 Chest Village

胸乡 *Xiong Xiang*

Effect Local effect on the *qi* in the channel, lowers it, frees the thorax.

Indications Pain laterally in the thorax that can also radiate into the back, cough, dyspnea. Point for self-sacrifice.

Localization In the third intercostal space on an imaginary contour line 1 cun below the height of the shoulder joint in the armpit.

Technique To a depth of about 0.3 cun; oblique insertion forward.

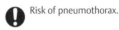 Risk of pneumothorax.

SP-20 All-Round Flourishing

周荣 *Zhou Rong*

Effect Local effect, regulates the flow of *qi*, transforms phlegm.

Indications Spasmodic cough with purulent sputum, dyspnea. Removes insecurity and emotional starvation, calms.

Localization In the second intercostal space on an imaginary contour line 1 cun below the height of the shoulder joint, barely accessible, deep inside the armpit.

Technique Barely accessible for needling.

 Risk of pneumothorax.

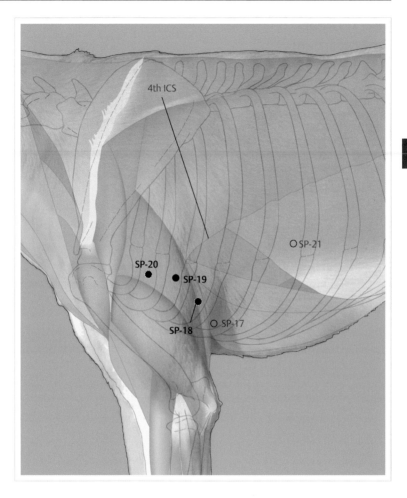

4th ICS

○ SP-21

SP-20

● SP-19

SP-18

○ SP-17

SP-21 Great Embracement

大包 *Da Bao*

Great connecting *luo*-point in the body.

Effect   Connects the sides of the body contralaterally, is connected to the *luo*-network vessels of other main channels via numerous smaller vessels, regulates *qi* and blood, frees the rib area.

Indications   Chest pain, intercostal neuralgia, lung disorders, generalized pain, weakness, pareses of the fore and hind paws. Concludes treatments by stabilizing; restores a sense of basic trust. In conjunction with HT-1, it is helpful in functional heart conditions caused by a blocked *qi* flow in the spleen channel.

Localization   Lateral on the thorax in the sixth intercostal space (although there are authors who have located it in the 10th intercostal space) on the height of an imaginary line connecting the shoulder and hip joints.

Technique   To a depth of about 0.3 cun; oblique insertion forward.

❗ Risk of pneumothorax.

SP

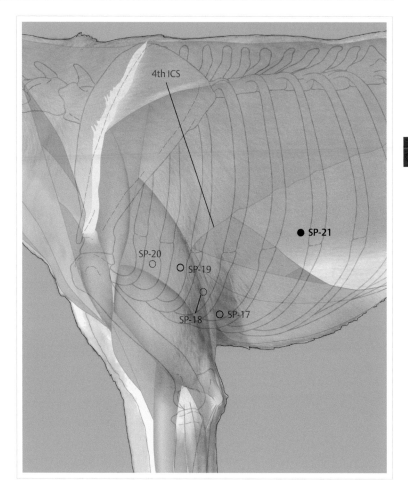

4th ICS

SP-21

SP-20

SP-19

SP-18

SP-17

15 Heart Channel

Hand *Shao Yin* (*Shou Shao Yin Xin Mai* 手少阴心脉)

The heart channel originates in the heart and the surrounding system of blood vessels (*xue mai*) and descends through the diaphragm to connect with the small intestine. One branch splits off in the heart and rises alongside the esophagus up to the face to connect with the tissue around the eyes. Another branch runs directly from the heart to the lung and surfaces in the armpit at the point HT-1. From there, the external heart channel runs along the medial upper arm to the elbow and along the caudolateral side of the forearm to the accessory bone, and from there palmar to the paw pad. From there, it runs between the fourth and fifth metacarpal bones to the medial nail fold of the fifth toe on the forefoot and ends there.

! The points on the heart channel must not be strongly stimulated because of their strong effect on the cardiovascular system.

HT

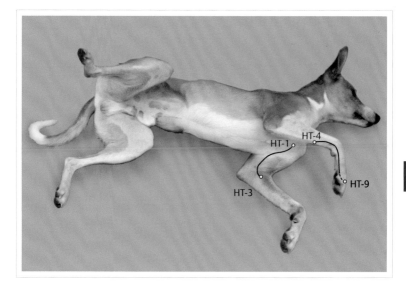

HT

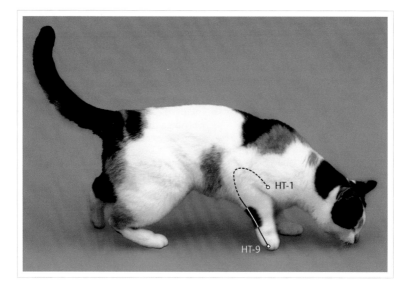

HT-1 Highest Spring
极泉 *Ji Quan*

Effect Is regarded as the most distal alarm point for the heart, diagnostic point, brings *qi* into the entire heart channel and increases it, makes the channel and network vessels passable.

Indications Pain in the thorax, dry cough, functional heart disorders, pain in the forelegs. For isolation due to an experience of shock.

Localization Deep in the center of the armpit, in the third intercostal space medial to the forelegs.

Technique To a maximum depth of 0.2 cun; tangential insertion along the rib line from the front to the back.

 Axillary plexus. Do not needle from lateral across the triceps, as there is risk of pneumothorax.

HT-2 Green-Blue Spirit
青灵 *Qing Ling*

Effect Makes the channel and network vessels passable, eliminates pain.

Indications Influential in regard to improved respiration, lateral thorax pain, shoulder and arm pain. Improves connection to *tian*.

Localization On the border of the lower third of the humerus on the medial edge of the biceps muscle of the arm.

Technique To a depth of 0.3 cun; perpendicular insertion, often recommended exclusively for moxibustion.

HT-3 Lesser Sea
少海 *Shao Hai*

He-sea point, water point.

Effect Removes obstructions in the channel, clears and calms the *shen*, eliminates phlegm and excess heat, stimulates the flow of heart *qi* and blood.

Indications Osteochondritis dissecans in the elbow joint, arthrosis/arthritis-related pain in the elbow joint, growth-related incongruence in the elbow joint, neuralgia of the ulnar nerve, psychological fatigue, epilepsy, fear, depression, psychologically caused lack of libido, increases the immune system defenses in infections, thoracic pain, and respiratory problems. Stabilizes and calms, to keep fears under control.

Localization Medial side of the forelegs, with the elbow flexed, in the middle between the end of the elbow flexion fold and the epicondyle of the humerus.

Technique To a depth of about 0.3 cun; perpendicular insertion.

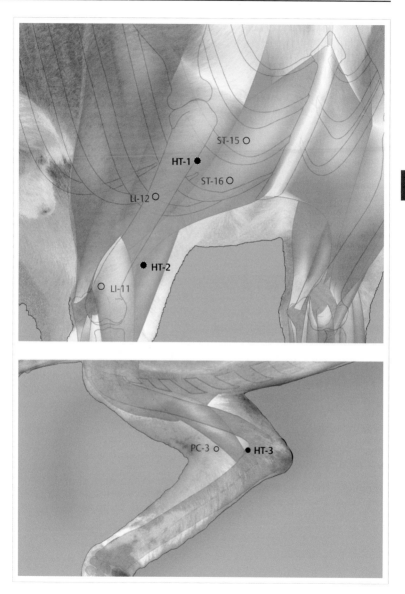

HT-4 Spirit Pathway
灵道 Ling Dao

Jing-river point, metal point.

Effect Nourishes the heart, strengthens and calms the *shen*, strengthens the voice, makes the network vessels passable.

Indications Improves circulation and stimulation in the muscle and tendon spindles of the flexor carpi ulnaris muscle; cardiovascular disorders; restlessness; pain in the paw, elbow, and forearm; states of anxiety; epilepsy; sleep disorders with vivid dreams; acute hoarseness/aphonia. For clouding of the senses due to suppressed pain.

Localization 2 cun above the accessory carpal bone, on the caudal edge of the flexor carpi ulnaris muscle.

Technique To a depth of about 0.3 cun; perpendicular insertion.

HT-5 Connecting *Li*
通里 Tong Li

Luo-network point.

Effect Calms the spirit, strengthens heart *qi*, supports the urinary bladder.

Indications Pain in the forelegs, contractions, spasms, pareses, circulatory disorders in the paws, tendency to tachycardia, hypertonicity, dizziness, urinary incontinence, urinary urgency upon excitement, sore throat, nausea, aerophagia, stage fright, claustrophobia. Autistic tendencies that cause shyness and reserved behavior or putting on a mask of happiness. Incongruent behavior.

Localization 1.5 cun above the accessory carpal bone, on the caudal edge of the flexor carpi ulnaris muscle.

Technique To a depth of about 0.3 cun; perpendicular insertion.

HT-6 *Yin* Cleft
阴郄 Yin Xi

Xi-cleft point.

Effect Calms the spirit, strengthens heart *yin* and heart blood, clears heart fire and deficiency of heat.

Indications Pain in the heart region, panting at night, states of fearful restlessness, dizziness, pain in the carpal joint. For hysteria without boundaries, and hyperactivity after trauma or shock.

Localization 1 cun above the accessory carpal bone, on the caudal edge of the flexor carpi ulnaris muscle.

Technique To a depth of about 0.3 cun; perpendicular insertion.

HT

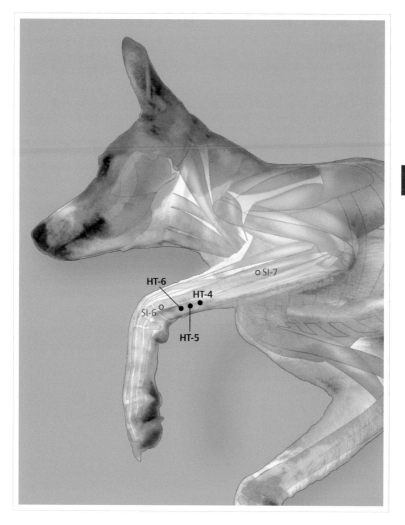

HT-7 Spirit Gate

神门 *Shen Men*

Yuan-source point, sedation point, *shu*-stream point, earth point.

Effect Calms the *shen* and the heart by strengthening heart blood and heart *yin*, resolves heart *qi* stagnation, frees the openings of the heart, clears heat and fire, clears the channels in the thorax.

HT

Indications Functional and organically caused heart problems (also due to psychological–physical strain), dry cough, respiratory complaints, general restlessness, irritability, nervousness, sleep disorders, depressive states, hysteria, urinary urgency, lack of energy, lack of appetite, vomiting, local point for pain in the forearm and carpal joint.

Localization Lateral, directly dorsal on the lower edge of the accessory carpal bone, in the transverse fold of the wrist when the carpal joint is flexed.

Technique To a depth of about 0.2 cun; perpendicular insertion.

HT-8 Lesser House

少府 *Shao Fu*

Ying-spring point, fire point.

Effect Eliminates deficiency of heat and phlegm heat as well as heart fire (main point), regulates heart *qi*, calms the spirit.

Indications Pain in the thorax and heart region; respiratory problems; restlessness; fear; psychoses that may lead to isolation; pain in the distal forelegs; fever; epilepsy; itching in the external genitals; dysuria; urinary retention; enuresis (extra point).

Localization Palmar surface of the paw. Between the fourth and fifth metacarpal bones in a dimple (palma manus) directly on the transition to the paw pad proximal to the metacarpophalangeal joint.

Technique To a depth of about 0.3 cun; perpendicular insertion.

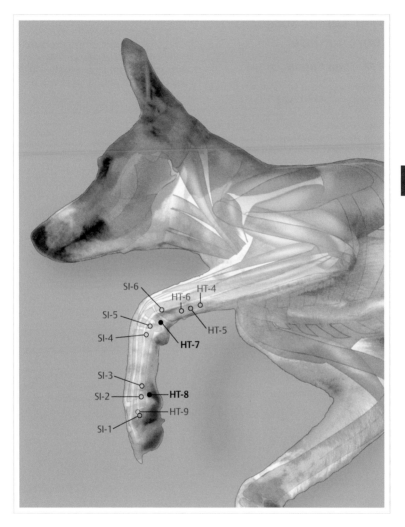

HT-9 Lesser Surge/ Thoroughfare

少冲 *Shao Chong*

Supplementing point for the heart channel, *jing*-well point, wood point.

Effect Eliminates heart heat, suppresses wind, frees the openings of the heart, relieves fullness, restores consciousness.

HT

Indications Psychological debility with excessive need for communication; fear; restlessness; melancholy; loss of libido; one of the most important points for emergencies such as shock, collapse, sunstroke, apoplexy, coma, etc.; heart and chest pain; contractions and pain on the inside of the forelegs; restlessness; arrhythmia; cardiac insufficiency; bradycardia; hypotonic states; catarrhs with hypersecretion in the bronchial tubes; lack of appetite; fever; distal point for all problems along the channel; pruritus of the vulva.

Localization Dorsally on the medial claw fold of the fifth toe of the forepaw directly above the proximal end of the claw.

Technique To a depth of about 0.2 cun; oblique insertion from below toward proximal.

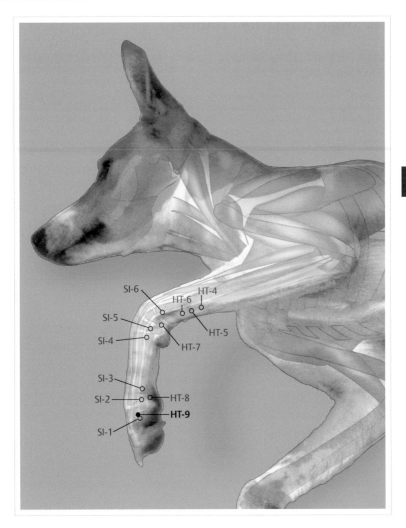

16 Small Intestine Channel

Hand *Tai Yang* (*Shou Tai Yang Xiao Chang Mai* 手太阳小肠脉)

The small intestine channel originates on the lateral side of the fifth fore toe and runs along the outside of the paw in a proximal direction. Shortly before the elbow, it briefly crosses over to the medial side of the elbow, then returns to the lateral side on the upper arm, and runs behind the shoulder joint to the point SI-10. It continues in a zigzag path across the scapula. From GV-14 on, the channel runs to the supraclavicular fossa and from there into the depth of the heart, continuing on along the esophagus in a caudal direction to the stomach. From there, it enters the small intestine.

Another branch continues from the supraclavicular fossa along the neck upward to the cheek, on to the lateral aspect of the eye, and from there to the ear. It runs around the ear and enters the ear at SI-19.

An additional branch descends from the small intestine to ST-39, the lower *he* point of the small intestine.

SI

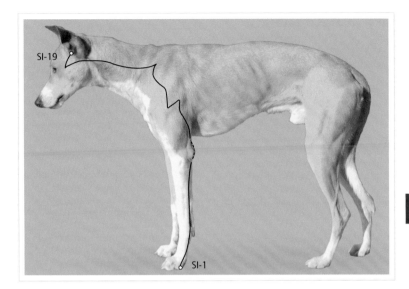

SI-19

SI-1

SI

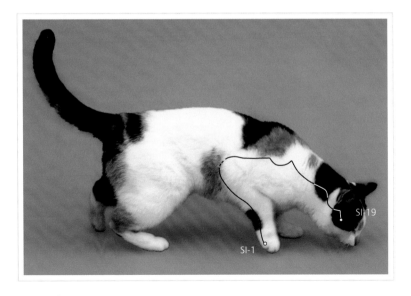

SI-1

SI-19

SI-1 Lesser Marsh
少泽 *Shao Ze*

Jing-well point, metal point.

Effect Expels wind-heat from the channel, frees the orifices, eliminates obstructions in the channel.

Indications Spasms of the forearm muscles, thorax pain, mastitis, deficient lactation, pharyngitis, laryngitis, exhaustion, torticollis, nausea, hyper- and hyposalivation, and visual defects; the point has a strong affinity with the mucous membranes. Helps with a more gentle integration of unknown traits.

Localization On the lateral claw fold of the fifth toe on the forepaw.

Technique To a depth of about 0.2 cun; oblique insertion upward.

SI-2 Front Valley
前谷 *Qian Gu*

Ying-brook point, water point.

Effect Draws out heat, moves *qi* along the channel.

Indications Pain in the forefoot and foreleg and in the neck and head area, mastitis, lack of lactation, colds and flu, nosebleeds, corneal clouding. Helps to strengthen confidence in one's own perceptions.

Localization Laterodistal to the base of the proximal phalanx of the fifth fore toe.

Technique To a depth of about 0.2 cun; perpendicular insertion.

SI-3 Back Ravine
后溪 *Hou Xi*

Shu-stream point, wood point, supplementing point, opener of the governing vessel (*du mai*), intersection point with the *yang* springing vessel (*yang qiao mai*).

Effect Draws internal wind out from the governing vessel (*du mai*) and small intestine channel, clears the channel, eliminates dampness, supports the tendons.

Indications Epilepsy, headache, pain in the neck and thoracic spine, shoulder pain, clears the throat, mastitis, agalactia, foreleg problems along the channel in combination with BL-62 to treat the entire back and neck, cramping in the paws, epilepsy, spasms, cramps in general, conditions resulting from stroke, helps the mucous membranes, conjunctivitis with tearing, blepharitis. Helps to distinguish between good and harmful.

Localization Proximal to the head of the fifth metacarpal bone, directly proximolateral to the metacarpophalangeal joint of the fifth fore toe.

Technique To a depth of about 0.3 cun; perpendicular insertion.

SI

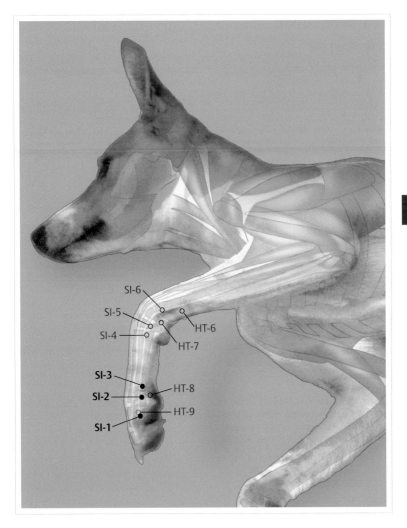

SI

SI-4 Wrist Bone

腕骨 *Wan Gu*

Yuan-source point.

Effect Clears damp-heat, activates the channel.

Indications Pain in the front toes and carpus, epicondylitis of the ulnar humerus, vomiting, tearing.

Localization Lateral on the carpal joint between the ulnar carpal bone and the base of the fifth metacarpal bone.

Technique To a depth of 0.2 cun; perpendicular insertion.

SI-5 *Yang* Valley

阳谷 *Yang Gu*

Jing-river point, fire point.

Effect Clears the *shen*, dispels external damp-heat, resolves obstructions in the channel.

Indications Pain and swelling in the carpus and in the neck and throat as well as the shoulder, jaw pain (dramatic), febrile disorders, meningeal irritation. Regulates in cases of withdrawal due to information overload.

Localization Lateral on the carpal joint between the ulnar carpal bone and the accessory carpal bone.

Technique To a depth of about 0.2 cun; perpendicular insertion.

SI-6 Nursing the Aged

养老 *Yang Lao*

Xi-cleft point.

Effect Supports the tendons, removes obstructions in the channel.

Indications Strong or acute pain in the upper joints of the forelegs, shoulder, and neck; stiffness in the back of the neck; hemiplegia; impaired vision; febrile disorders. Helps with the digestion of unprocessed experiences.

Localization Proximolateral directly above the carpus, slightly radial to the tip of the styloid process of the ulna.

Technique To a depth of about 0.3 cun; perpendicular insertion.

SI

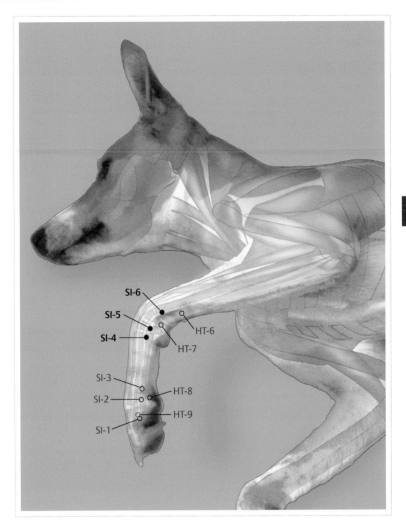

SI-7 Branch to the Correct

支正 *Zhi Zheng*

Luo-network point.

Effect Affects the small intestine directly via the longitudinal *luo*-network vessel, clears heat and frees the surface, eliminates obstructions in the channel.

Indications Pain in the toes and paws, spasms of the forearm muscles, fever, stiff neck, alternating irritability and apathy, tendency to tachycardia with fearfulness, inflammations in the jaw, intestinal colics, obstipation.

Localization Caudolateral in the middle (cranial edge) of the forearm on the belly of the extensor carpi ulnaris muscle.

Technique To a depth of about 1 cun; perpendicular insertion.

SI-8 Small Sea

小海 *Xiao Hai*

He-sea point, earth point, sedation point.

Effect Eliminates damp-heat and obstructions in the channel, calms the spirit.

Indications Acute swelling of the glands in the back of the neck and throat, neuralgia or paralysis of the ulnar nerve, all elbow problems (osteochondrosis dissecans, incongruence), shoulder and neck pain, epilepsy, hearing loss, toothache and gingivitis, lower abdominal pain. For involuntary movements. Imparts emotional stability.

Localization Medial on the elbow, between the medial epicondyle of the humerus and the olecranon, about 1 cun from the tip of the olecranon.

Technique To a depth of about 0.2 cun; almost perpendicular insertion, slightly toward cranial.

SI-9 True Shoulder

肩真 *Jian Zhen*

Effect Moves *qi* along the course of the channel, eliminates wind.

Indications Shoulder joint pain and pain in the area of the shoulder blade, elbow pain, analgesia.

Localization Caudomedial to the humerus in a large depression along the posterior edge of the deltoid muscle, where it connects to the lateral head of the triceps muscle of the arm.

Technique To a depth of 0.5 cun; perpendicular insertion from the inside outward.

SI

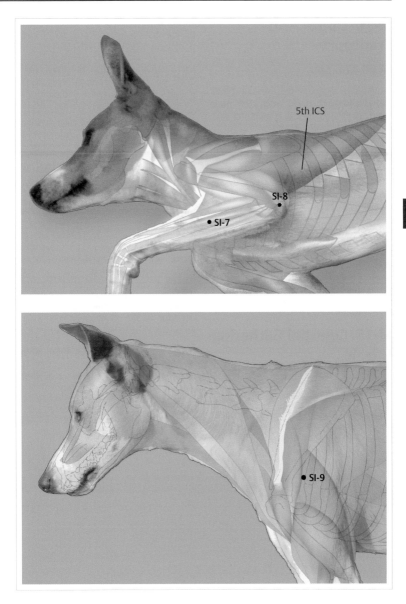

SI

SI-10 Upper Arm Transport

臑俞 *Nao Shu*

Intersection point of the small intestine and bladder channels with the *yang springing vessel* (*yang qiao mai*) and *yang linking vessel* (*yang wei mai*).

Effect Removes painful obstructions in the channel.

Indications Pain and weakness in the neck and shoulder area, cramps in the paws.

Localization Directly on the posterior edge of the shoulder joint on the deltoid muscle, on the acromial part from the lateral side.

Technique To a depth of about 0.5 to 1 cun; perpendicular insertion.

SI-11 Celestial Gathering

天宗 *Tian Zong*

Effect Moves *qi* along the course of the channel, frees the thorax.

Indications Pain in the area of the cheek and chin, neck, shoulders, and forelegs; impaired ability to move the forelegs backward; swelling and lateral deviation of the shoulder; mammary pain during lactation. Helps in getting rid of perfectionism.

Localization Central in the infraspinous fossa on the infraspinous and deltoid muscles, directly above the acromion.

Technique To a depth of about 1.5 cun; perpendicular insertion.

SI-12 Grasping the Wind

秉风 *Bing Feng*

Intersection point of the small intestine, large intestine, triple burner, and gallbladder channels.

Effect Moves *qi* along the course of the channel, eliminates wind.

Indications Impaired ability to bring the forelegs backward, swelling and lateral deviation of the shoulder, tension in the dorsal neck due to lack of purpose.

Localization In the lower third of the supraspinous fossa at the height of the acromion and SI-11 on the supraspinous and omotransversarius muscles.

Technique To a depth of about 1.5 cun; perpendicular insertion.

SI

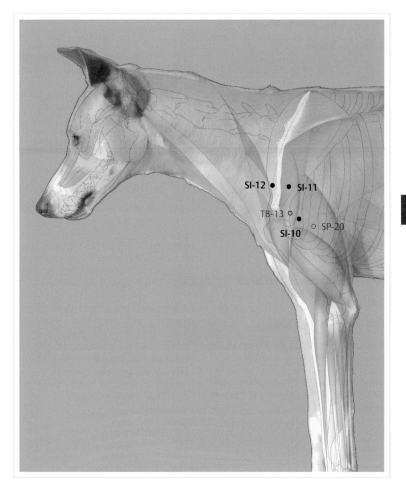

SI-13 Crooked Wall
曲垣 *Qu Yuan*

Effect   Moves *qi* along the course of the channel.

Indications   Painful muscle contractions in the shoulder area, swelling and lateral deviation of the shoulder.

Localization   Lateral on the cranial border of the scapula above SI-12 and in the angle between the lower edge of the cervical part of the trapezius muscle and the omo-transversarius muscle.

Technique   To a depth of about 1.5 cun; perpendicular insertion.

SI-14 Outer Shoulder Transport
肩外俞 *Jian Wai Shu*

Effect   Moves *qi* along the course of the channel, eliminates wind and cold.

Indications   Pain in the shoulder joint and shoulder blade, scleroses in the neck and withers.

Localization   At the height of the cranial angle of the scapula on the upper end of the anterior edge of the scapula, on the transition from bone to cartilage, lateral to the first thoracic vertebra.

Technique   To a depth of about 1 cun; oblique insertion from lateral upward.

SI-15 Central Shoulder Transport
肩中俞 *Jian Zhong Shu*

Effect   Moves *qi* along the course of the channel, helps in lowering lung *qi*.

Indications   Pain in the shoulder blade, swelling in the shoulder joint, pain and scleroses in the neck and withers, cough, dyspnea. Opens up unclear perception.

Localization   Cranial to SI-14 in the pre-scapular groove, lateral to the lower edge of the seventh cervical vertebra.

Technique   To a depth of about 1.5 cun; perpendicular insertion.

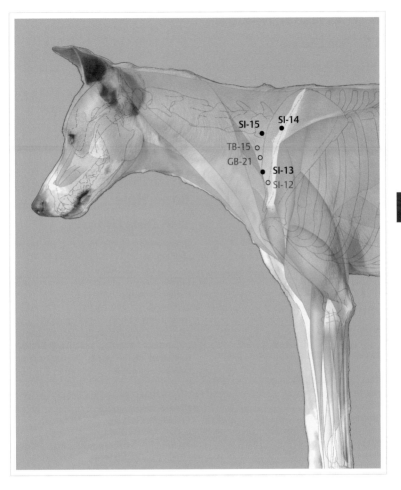

SI-15

SI-14

TB-15

GB-21

SI-13

SI-12

SI-16 Celestial Window
天窗 *Tian Chuang*

Effect Moves *qi* along the course of the channel; clears heat; supports the ears, neck, and voice.

Indications Neck pain, pain and scleroses in the withers, torticollis, swelling in the flews, struma, sudden loss of voice or deafness, excessive cleanliness.

Localization On the dorsal edge of the mastoid part of the cleidocephalicus muscle between the transverse processes of the second and third cervical vertebrae.

Technique To a depth of about 1 cun; perpendicular insertion.

SI-17 Celestial Countenance
天容 *Tian Rong*

Union point with the gallbladder channel.

Effect Lowers rebellious *qi*; supports the neck, throat, and ears.

Indications Cough, dyspnea, swollen flews, any form of inflammation in the neck and throat, struma.

Localization In a depression between the corner of the jaw and the cranial edge of the sternocleidomastoid muscle, above the carotid artery, jugular vein, and cranial cervical ganglion.

Technique To a depth of about 0.5 cun; perpendicular insertion.

 Blood vessels and nerve tissue.

SI-18 Influential Bone-Hole
权髎 *Quan Liao*

Intersection point with the triple burner channel.

Effect Draws out wind, clears heat, reduces swelling.

Indications Facial nerve paralysis, trigeminal neuralgia of the second branch, infraorbital swelling, maxillary sinusitis, toothache in the upper jaw; for calming down.

Localization Below the lateral corner of the eye, ventral to the temporal process of the zygomatic bone.

Technique To a depth of about 0.2 cun; perpendicular insertion.

SI

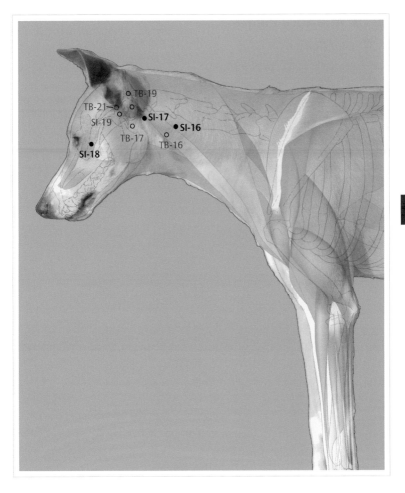

SI-19 Auditory Palace

听宫 *Ting Gong*

Intersection point of the small intestine, triple burner, and gallbladder channels.

Effect   Stimulates all *yang* channels, calms the spirit.

Indications   Otitis external, otitis media, arthritis of the temporomandibular joint, laryngitis, deafness, epilepsy. Improves the ability to focus on what is essential.

Localization   In front of the ear, caudal to the mandible, rostral to the tragus, directly ventral to TB-21, slightly dorsal to the condyles when the mouth is open.

 Mnemonic verse for the three points located underneath each other on the ear. TB-21 on top, SI-19 in the middle, GB-2 below (2 + 19 = 21).

Technique   To a depth of about 0.3 cun; perpendicular insertion.

SI

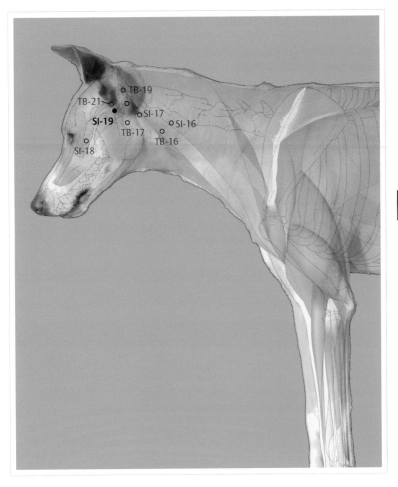

17 Bladder Channel

Foot *Tai Yang* (*Zu Tai Yang Pang Guang Mai* 足太阳膀胱脉)

The bladder channel starts by the eye. From the medial canthus at BL-1, it ascends across the forehead. From there, a branch runs to the temples. Another branch enters the brain from the forehead, and then meets up with GV-17 where it exits to the surface, and splits into the internal and external bladder channels in the vicinity of BL-10. These run parallel on both sides of the spine in a caudal direction.

The medial branch descends across the back of the neck, meets up with GV-14 and GV-13, and runs lateral to the midline all the way to the lumbar area. From there, a branch runs deep inside to the bladder and kidney, and another branch runs along the sacrum across the croup to the knee fold and the point BL-40.

The external bladder channel runs along the medial border of the scapula and then parallel to the midline, lateral to the internal bladder channel, all the way to the gluteal area, crosses GB-30, and meets up with the internal bladder channel at BL-40. From the popliteal fold, the reunited bladder channel runs through the gastrocnemius muscle distal to the lateral part of the tarsus, to end at the lateral nail fold of the fifth toe of the hind paw.

BL

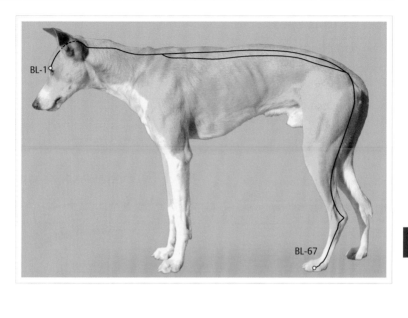

BL-1

BL-67

BL

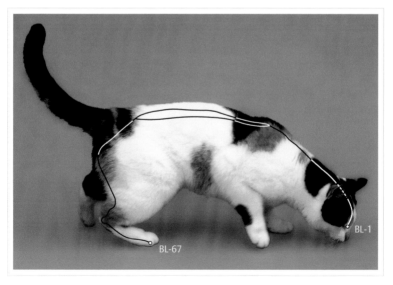

BL-67

BL-1

BL-1 Bright Eyes

睛明 *Jing Ming*

Intersection point of the bladder, small intestine, stomach, gallbladder, and triple burner channels, the governing vessel (*du mai*), and the *yin* and *yang* springing vessels (*yin qiao mai* and *yang qiao mai*).

Effect   Expels wind, clears heat, and clears the eyes.

Indications   Conjunctivitis, keratitis, cataracts, supporting point for atrophy of the optic nerve, tearing with exposure to wind, trigeminal neuralgia; for calming and brightening the mood.

Localization   0.1 cun nasal to the medial canthus.

Technique   To a depth of 0.3 cun; slightly oblique insertion downward from above.

 Do not stimulate.

BL-2 Bamboo Gathering

攢竹 *Zan Zhu*

Effect   Expels wind, stops pain, eliminates obstructions in the channel, clears the eyes, calms *gan.*

Indications   Eye disorders such as conjunctivitis, keratitis; frontal sinusitis; constant sneezing (depending on the cause, also so-called "reverse sneezing"); trigeminal neuralgia; for calming.

Localization   On the medial end of the eyebrow, on the nasal edge of the orbit, dorsal to BL-1.

Technique   To a depth of about 0.1 cun; perpendicular insertion.

BL-3 Eyebrow Ascension

眉冲 *Mei Chong*

Effect   Moves *qi* along the course of the channel, draws out wind, supports the eyes and nose.

Indications   Eye disorders with swelling of the eyelids, frontal sinusitis, epileptiform seizures, lesions on the nose. Weakens fears by making them conscious.

Localization   0.5 cun lateral to the midline, roughly halfway on the external frontal crest.

Technique   To a depth of about 0.1 cun; perpendicular insertion.

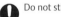 Do not stimulate.

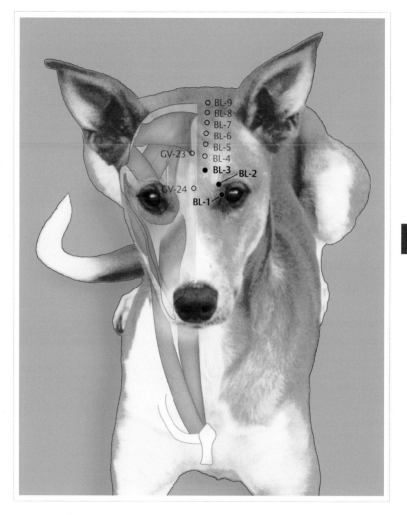

BL

BL-4 Deviating Turn

曲差 *Qu Cha*

Effect Moves *qi* along the course of the channel, draws out wind, supports the eyes and nose.

Indications Conjunctivitis, rhinitis, blepharitis, sinusitis, lesions on the nose.

Localization 0.5 cun lateral to the midline, on a sagittal line with BL-2 at the height of the rostral edge of the ear, caudal to the external frontal crest.

Technique To a depth of about 0.1 cun; perpendicular insertion.

BL-5 Fifth Place

五处 *Wu Chu*

Effect Draws out wind, eliminates heat, brings down *yang*, clears the head.

Indications Epileptiform seizures, spasms, stiffness in the spine, calms panic attacks.

Localization On a sagittal line with BL-2 to BL-7, in a caudal direction.

Technique To a depth of about 0.1 cun; perpendicular insertion.

BL-6 Light Guard

承光 *Cheng Guang*

Effect Draws out wind, clears heat, clears the head, supports the eyes and nose.

Indications Pain in the head and eyes, dizziness, nausea, facial nerve paresis, impaired sense of smell, depression.

Localization On a sagittal line with BL-2 to BL-7.

Technique To a depth of about 0.1 cun; perpendicular insertion.

BL-7 Celestial Connection

通天 *Tong Tian*

Effect Supports the nose, clears the head.

Indications Cervical syndrome, rhinitis, sinusitis, being flooded with fear.

Localization 0.5 cun lateral to the midline at the level of the ear canal.

Technique To a depth of about 0.1 cun; tangential insertion.

BL

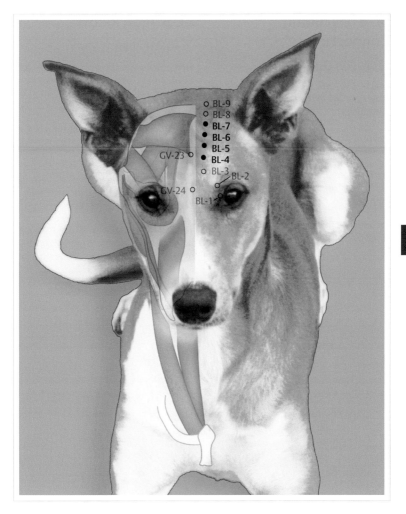

BL-8 Declining Connection

络却 *Luo Que*

Effect Supports the eyes, ears, and nose, draws out wind, calms the spirit, transforms phlegm.

Indications Rhinitis, epistaxis, cervical syndrome, jaw problems, struma.

Localization Halfway between BL-7 and BL-9 on a sagittal line slightly lateral to the midline.

Technique To a depth of about 0.1 cun; tangential insertion.

BL-9 Jade Pillow

玉枕 *Yu Zhen*

Effect Supports the nose and eyes, conducts *qi* from there to the brain, draws out wind and cold, resolves obstructions in the channel.

Indications Rhinitis, loss of the sense of smell, cervical syndrome, jaw problems. Brings clarity to fears.

Localization On the temporal crest, lateral to the midline, on a line with BL-3 to BL-8.

Technique To a depth of about 0.1 cun; perpendicular insertion.

BL

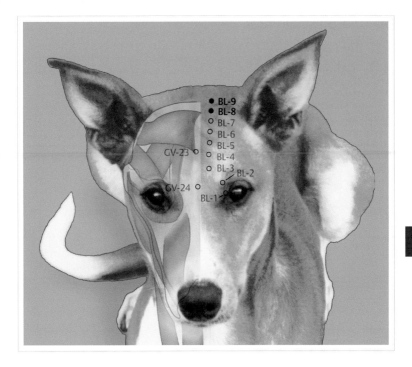

BL

BL-10 Celestial Pillar

天柱 *Tian Zhu*

Effect Expels wind, clears the eyes, supports the head, removes obstructions from the channel.

Indications Localized problems such as cervical syndrome, shoulder, back; strengthens the lumbar spine; helps with problems of the contralateral hind leg, intervertebral disks, and spondyloses; eye disorders; encephalitis; torticollis; lowers blood pressure ("vagus point"); arteriosclerosis. Connects head and emotions.

Localization Between the first and second cervical vertebrae, on the posterior edge of the wing of the atlas, 1.5 cun lateral, on the origin of the trapezius muscle, behind which the bladder channel separates into the internal and external branches.

Technique To a depth of about 1 cun; perpendicular insertion.

BL

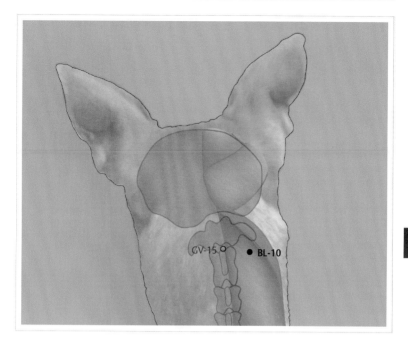

BL-11 Great Shuttle

大杼 *Da Zhu*

Intersection point of the bladder, small intestine, and triple burner channels, the controlling vessel (*ren mai*) and governing vessel (*du mai*), master point of the bones, one point of the sea of blood.

Effect Strengthens the *qi*, eliminates wind and pathogenic factors, nourishes the blood, relieves pain, nourishes the tendons, stabilizes the bone structure, heals bone tissue.

Indications All bone diseases, also of a degenerative nature; pain in the neck, back, and forelegs; problems with the respiratory tract; fever; arthrosis; problems with the cervical disks. Creates perseverance, having the guts to do something.

Localization 1.5 cun lateral to the posterior edge of the spinous process of the first thoracic vertebra, halfway between the spinous process and the medial edge of the scapula.

Technique To a depth of about 1 cun; perpendicular insertion.

 Risk of pneumothorax.

BL-12 Wind Gate

风门 *Feng Men*

Intersection point of the bladder channel and the governing vessel (*du mai*).

Effect Dispels wind, opens and strengthens the surface, supports the lung's function of distributing and lowering *qi*.

Indications Problems of the respiratory tract and trachea; bronchitis; asthma; sneezing; pain in the throat, scapula, and back; itching, possibly with urticaria.

Localization 1.5 cun lateral to the posterior edge of the spinous process of the second thoracic vertebra.

Technique To a depth of about 1 cun; perpendicular insertion.

 Risk of pneumothorax.

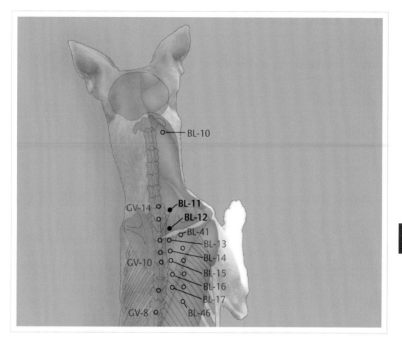

BL-13 Lung Transport

肺俞 *Fei Shu*

Effect Supports the lung's function of distributing and lowering *qi*, regulates and strengthens lung *qi*, quietens coughing, eliminates heat.

Indications Common cold; bronchitis; fever; respiratory tract problems, also chronic ones; problems of the medial extremities; pruritic dermatitis.

Localization 1.5 cun lateral to the posterior edge of the spinous process of the third thoracic vertebra.

Technique To a depth of about 1 cun; perpendicular insertion.

 Risk of pneumothorax.

BL-14 Reverting *Yin* Transport

厥阴俞 *Jue Yin Shu*

Effect Balances and lowers *qi*, distributes liver *qi* and frees the thorax, regulates the heart.

Indications Anxiety; respiratory tract problems; cold with fever; problems of the forelegs; problems and pain in the chest, ribs, sternum, myocarditis, pericarditis.

Localization 1.5 cun lateral to the posterior edge of the spinous process of the fourth thoracic vertebra.

Technique To a depth of about 1 cun; perpendicular insertion.

 Risk of pneumothorax.

BL-15 Heart Transport

心俞 *Xin Shu*

Effect Supports the heart, calms the spirit, quickens the blood, regulates the circulation of *qi* and *xue*, clears heat-related fire.

Indications Cardiac problems, anxiety, pain in the area of the shoulder blades, epilepsy.

Localization 1.5 cun lateral to the posterior edge of the spinous process of the fifth thoracic vertebra.

Technique To a depth of about 1 cun; perpendicular insertion.

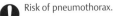 Risk of pneumothorax.

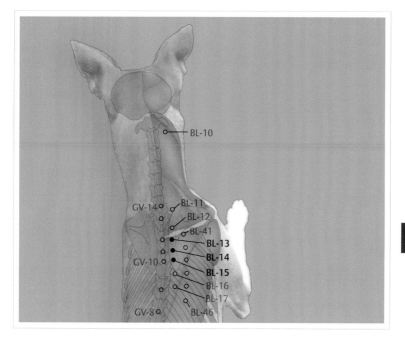

BL-16 Governing Transport

督俞 *Du Shu*

Effect Quickens the blood (*xue*).

Indications Myocarditis, pericarditis, back pain, abdominal pain, pruritic skin disorders.

Localization 1.5 cun lateral to the posterior edge of the spinous process of the sixth thoracic vertebra.

Technique To a depth of about 1 cun; perpendicular insertion.

 Risk of pneumothorax.

BL-17 Diaphragm Transport

膈俞 *Ge Shu*

Effect Influential point for the diaphragm, respiration, and the blood. Lowers rebellious *qi*, nourishes and quickens the blood, cools blood heat, stanches bleeding, opens the thorax, strengthens *qi* and blood, regulates stomach *qi*.

Indications Strengthens the blood and the immune system in hemorrhages, for all blood disorders, problems in the thorax and its organs, regulates the pancreas, esophageal spasms, generalized pain.

Localization 1.5 cun lateral to the posterior edge of the spinous process of the seventh thoracic vertebra.

Technique To a depth of about 1 cun; perpendicular insertion.

 Risk of pneumothorax.

BL-18 Liver Transport

肝俞 *Gan Shu*

Effect Strengthens the liver's function of promoting harmonious *qi* flow, nourishes the liver and blood, disperses and transforms dampness and heat from the gallbladder (*dan*) and liver (*gan*), clears the eyes, brightens the gaze, expels wind.

Indications Problems related to muscle function; problems of the tendons, stomach, eye, liver, and gallbladder; hormonal disturbances; strengthens the immune system; pain in the upper body.

Localization 1.5 cun lateral to the posterior edge of the spinous process of the 10th thoracic vertebra.

Technique To a depth of about 1 cun; perpendicular insertion.

 Risk of pneumothorax.

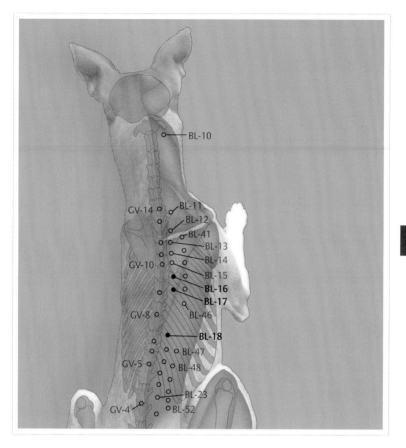

BL-19 Gallbladder Transport

胆俞 *Dan Shu*

Effect Strengthens the liver's function of promoting harmonious *qi* flow, disperses and transforms dampness and heat from *dan* and *gan*, eliminates pathogenic factors from the triple burner and gallbladder channels, *shao yang*, calms the stomach.

Indications Problems along the channel; problems of the tendons and muscles, brain, stomach; pain in the lateral rib area.

Localization 1.5 cun lateral to the posterior edge of the spinous process of the 11th thoracic vertebra.

Technique To a depth of about 1 cun; perpendicular insertion.

 Risk of pneumothorax.

BL-20 Spleen Transport

脾俞 *Pi Shu*

Effect Strengthens the spleen's function of transformation and transport, strengthens the spleen's (*pi*) function of upwardly directed flow of *qi*, disperses and transforms dampness.

Indications Problems along the channel, problems of the medial knee, bleeding, stomach problems, digestive complaints, problems with the pancreas, edemas, ascites, aid in obstetric problems, stimulate the immune system.

Localization 1.5 cun lateral to the posterior edge of the spinous process of the 12th thoracic vertebra (last intercostal space).

Technique To a depth of about 1 cun; perpendicular insertion.

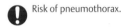 Risk of pneumothorax.

BL-21 Stomach Transport

胃俞 *Wei Shu*

Effect Strengthens the stomach's (*wei*) function of moving *qi* downward, resolves colic pain, disperses and transforms dampness, resolves stagnation in the stomach.

Indications Problems of the lateral knee, stomach problems, vomiting, colic, digestive disorders.

Localization 1.5 cun lateral to the posterior edge of the spinous process of the 13th thoracic vertebra.

Technique To a depth of about 1 cun; perpendicular insertion.

 Risk of pneumothorax.

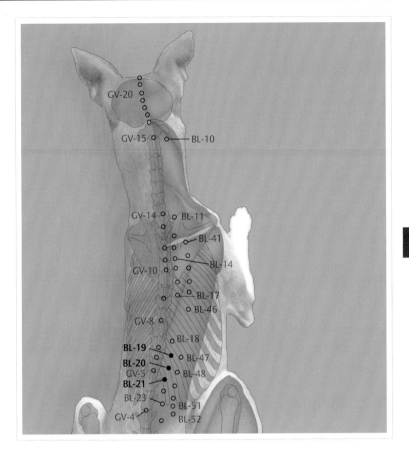

BL-22 Triple Burner Transport
三焦俞 *San Jiao Shu*

Effect Regulates the transformative functions of *qi*, disperses dampness, opens the waterways, regulates the transport of fluids in the lower burner. (The triple burner is important for endocrine imbalances of the thyroid and adrenal glands and gonads and the corresponding emotional problems.) It regulates the stomach, as well as pain and stiffness in the lower back.

Indications Digestive disorders, dysentery, gastrointestinal spasms, lumbago, nephritis, edemas, ascites, endocrine disorders, abdominal distention with emaciation, localized intervertebral disk problems.

Localization 1.5 cun lateral to the caudal edge of the spinous process of the first lumbar vertebra.

Technique To a depth of about 1 cun; perpendicular insertion.

BL-23 Kidney Transport
肾俞 *Shen Shu*

Effect Supplements kidney *yin* and the essence; strengthens the marrow, bones, and ears; disperses and resolves dampness; strengthens the kidney's function of regulating the waterways; strengthens kidney *yang* and *qi*; opens the waterways; supports and warms the uterus; regulates the transport of fluids in the lower burner; strengthens the lower back and knees.

Indications Urogenital and lumbosacral problems, asthma, problems with the ankle, ear problems, nephritis, ovarian problems, andrological problems, reproductive disorders, pain in the hip, cold or paralysis in the hind legs, polyuria, chronic diarrhea.

Localization 1.5 cun lateral to the caudal edge of the spinous process of the second lumbar vertebra.

Technique To a depth of about 1 cun; perpendicular insertion.

BL-24 Sea of *Qi* Transport
气海俞 *Qi Hai Shu*

Effect Strengthens the lower back, regulates *qi* and blood, removes obstructions.

Indications Pain in the lumbosacral area, fatigue, listlessness, weakened immune system.

Localization 1.5 cun lateral to the ventral spinous process of the third lumbar vertebra.

Technique To a depth of about 1 cun; perpendicular insertion.

BL

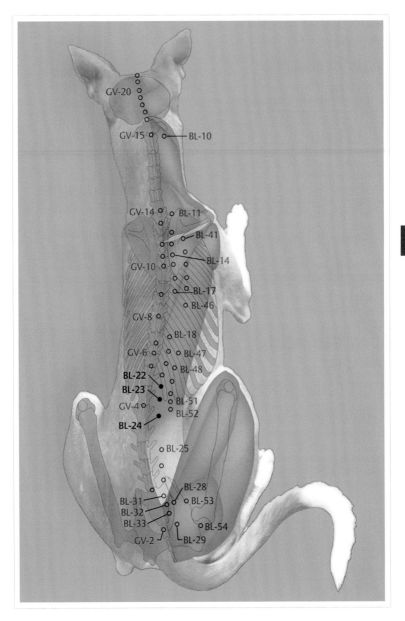

BL-25 Large Intestine Transport

大肠俞 *Da Chang Shu*

Effect Supports the transport function of the intestine, relieves fullness and abdominal distention, strengthens the lumbar region and sacrum, removes obstructions from the channel.

Indications Pain in the face, mouth, back of the neck, shoulder, and in the lateral area of the foreleg; pain in the lower back and hip; ischial complaints; gastrointestinal problems; colic; obstipation; enteritis; diarrhea; tenesmus, problems of the rectum and anus; fever; rhinitis; dyspnea.

Localization 1.5 cun lateral to the ventral spinous process of the fifth lumbar vertebra.

Technique To a depth of about 1 cun; perpendicular insertion.

BL-26 Pass Head Transport

关元俞 *Guan Yuan Shu*

Effect Regulates the lower burner, infertility, retained placenta, kidney and bladder problems, rectal prolapse.

Indications Lumbago, intestinal spasms, edemas in the genital area, digestive problems, diarrhea, endometriosis, support during hormone therapy, urinary incontinence, cystitis, problems in the iliosacral joint.

Localization 1 cun lateral to the ventral spinous process of the sixth lumbar vertebra.

Technique To a depth of about 1 cun; perpendicular insertion.

BL-27 Small Intestine Transport

小肠俞 *Xiao Chang Shu*

Effect Draws out turbid dampness and clears damp-heat, regulates the abdominal organs and bladder, removes stagnation and disperses masses.

Indications Pain in the posterior back, digestive problems, ischialgia, pain in the lower abdomen, andropathies, impotence, obstetric complications, urinary problems, incontinence, urethritis, cystitis.

Localization 1 cun lateral to the ventral spinous process of the seventh lumbar spine by the beginning of the sacrum.

Technique To a depth of about 1 cun; perpendicular insertion.

 Contraindicated during pregnancy.

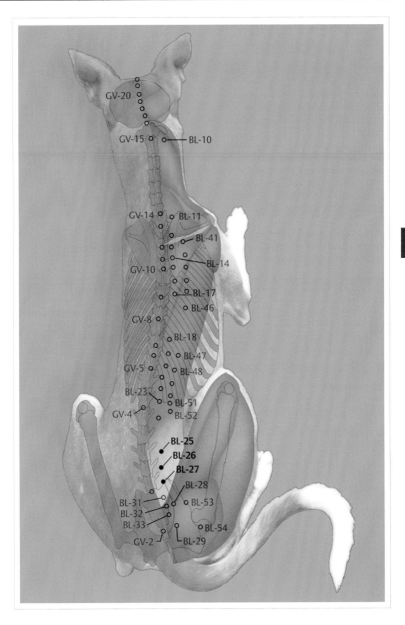

BL-28 Bladder Transport
膀胱俞 *Pang Guan Shu*

Effect Strengthens kidney *yang*, regulates the passage of water in the lower burner, eliminates dampness, clears heat, supports the functions of the urinary and reproductive systems, eliminates obstructions in the channel.

Indications Stiffness and pain in the neck and back; cauda equina syndrome; problems in the urogenital tract; weakened genitals, libido, and reproduction; abdominal pain; colic; coughing; colds.

Localization Lateral to the second sacral foramen, in a depression between the medial edge of the dorsal ilium and the sacrum.

Technique To a depth of about 1 cun; perpendicular insertion.

 Contraindicated during pregnancy.

BL-29 Central Backbone Transport
中膂俞 *Zhong Lü Shu*

Effect Supports the back, expels cold, checks diarrhea.

Indications Stiffness and pain in the lower back in the lumbar and sacral regions, cauda equina syndrome, proctitis, enterocolitis, urinary tract disorders, urinary problems, gynecological problems, andrological problems, impotence, problems of the rectum and anus.

Localization At the level of the sacrococcygeal space between the sacrum and the first coccygeal vertebra on a line between the ischiadic tuber and the dorsal cranial iliac spine.

Technique To a depth of about 1 cun; perpendicular insertion.

BL-30 White Ring Transport
白环俞 *Bai Huan Shu*

Owing to the reduced number of sacral vertebrae in dogs and cats compared with humans, BL-30 is not extant.

BL

BL

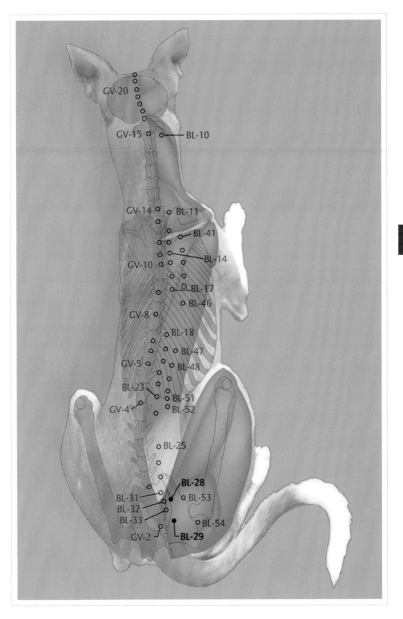

BL-31–BL-34 Eight Bone-Holes

八髎 *Ba Liao*

BL-31 Upper Bone-Hole

上髎 *Shang Liao*

Union point with the gallbladder channel at GB-30.

Effect Regulates the lower burner, nourishes the kidneys, promotes *jing* essence, supplements the lumbar region and knees.

Indications Pain and edemas in the hind leg, paralysis in the hip and penis, cauda equina syndrome, problems in the iliosacral joint, infertility due to changes in the cervix.

Localization 0.5 cun lateral to the midline, above the first sacral foramen, dorsomedial to BL-27.

Technique To a depth of about 0.5 cun; perpendicular insertion.

BL-32 Second Bone-Hole

次髎 *Ci Liao*

Union point with the gallbladder channel at GB-30.

Effect Regulates the lower burner, nourishes the kidneys, promotes *jing* essence, supplements the lumbar region and knees.

Indications Pain and edemas in the hind leg, paralysis in the hip and penis, cauda equina syndrome, problems in the iliosacral joint, infertility due to changes in the cervix, vaginal problems.

Localization 0.5 cun lateral to the midline, above the second sacral foramen, dorsomedial to BL-28.

Technique To a depth of about 0.5 cun; perpendicular insertion.

BL-33 Third Bone-Hole

中髎 *Zhong Liao*

Union point with the gallbladder channel at GB-30.

Effect Regulates the lower burner, nourishes the kidneys, promotes *jing* essence, supplements the lumbar region and knees, facilitates urination and defecation.

Indications Pain in the lower back, pain and edemas in the hind leg, paralysis in the hip and penis, cauda equina syndrome, problems in the iliosacral joint, irregular estrous cycle, diarrhea, constipation, more influence on the bladder.

Localization 0.5 cun lateral to the midline, above the second sacral foramen, dorsomedial to BL-29.

Technique To a depth of about 0.5 cun; perpendicular insertion.

BL

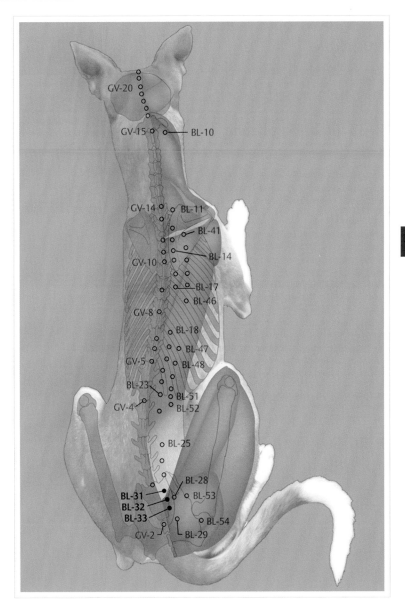

BL

BL-34 Lower Bone-Hole
下髎 *Xia Liao*

Owing to the reduced number of sacral vertebrae in dogs and cats compared with humans, BL-34 is not extant.

BL-35 Meeting of *Yang*
会阳 *Hui Yang*

Effect Moves *qi* locally in the anal region and in the lower colon as well as in the lower spine, clears damp-heat.

Indications Anal gland inflammation; vaginitis; orchitis; diarrhea; rectal prolapse; hip joint arthritis; myositis in the muscles of the hind leg; paralysis in the loins, sciatic nerve, femoral nerve, and penis; vaginal and cervical problems; paresis or paralysis in the hind legs.

Localization In the muscle channel lateral to the base of the tail, 0.5 cun lateral to the governing vessel, localized by lifting the tail, at the height of the transition from the first to second coccygeal vertebra.

Technique To a depth of about 0.5 cun; perpendicular insertion.

BL-36 Support
承扶 *Cheng Fu*

Local point, diagnostic point for the hip.

Effect Activates the channel and relaxes the tendons.

Indications Impaired movement in the hind leg, pelvic rotation, hip joint luxation, myositis in the biceps femoris, ischialgia, lumbago, rectal prolapse, anal sac inflammation, prostate problems, testicular and vaginal disorders. Is helpful for the feeling that one has to carry all the weight by oneself.

Localization In the muscle channel between the biceps femoris and semitendinous muscle, directly ventral to the tuberosity of the ischium.

Technique To a depth of about 1 cun; perpendicular insertion.

BL-37 Gate of Abundance
殷门 *Yin Men*

Effect Activates the channel and resolves obstructions in its course.

Indications Lameness in the hind leg, lumbago, gonitis, pelvic rotation, hip joint luxation, myositis of the biceps femoris, ischialgia.

Localization In the muscle channel between the biceps femoris and semitendinous muscle, 3 cun ventral to BL-36, in the middle of an imaginary line from BL-36 to BL-40.

Technique To a depth of about 1 cun; perpendicular insertion.

BL

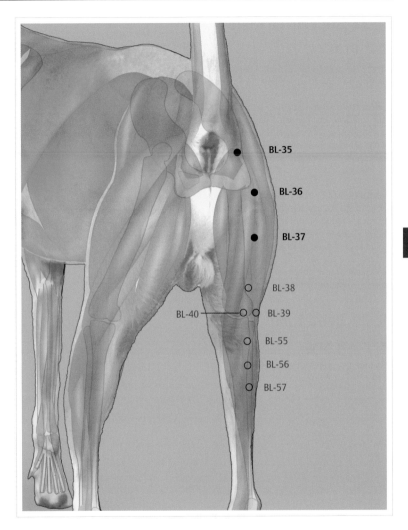

BL-35
BL-36
BL-37

BL

BL-38
BL-40 ——— BL-39
BL-55
BL-56
BL-57

BL-38 Superficial Cleft

浮郄 *Fu Xi*

Effect Resolves obstructions along the channel, prevents contractions, clears heat.

Indications Muscle spasms, paralysis and pain laterally on the hind legs, gonitis, gonarthrosis, pelvic rotation, myositis of the biceps femoris, problems with the sciatic nerve, cystitis, hemorrhaging (bleeding), obstipation.

Localization In the muscle channel between the biceps femoris, medial to its terminal tendon and the semitendinous muscle, 3 cun ventral to BL-37, proximolateral to the hollow of the knee.

Technique To a depth of about 1 cun; perpendicular insertion.

BL-39 Bend *Yang*

委阳 *Wei Yang*

Lower *he*-sea point of the lower burner.

Effect Diagnostic point for the ankle; excess of fluids (*jin ye*), especially in the lower burner; opens the waterways; supports the bladder; for excess in the lower burner.

Indications Lameness and pain in the hind leg and tarsus, disturbances in the urogenital tract, cystitis, urinary problems, urinary retention, colic of the kidney and urinary tract, for stubbornness.

Localization Lateral to the popliteal fold on the medial edge of the terminal tendon of the biceps femoris, directly lateral to BL-40, in a depression in the end of the channel between the biceps femoris and semitendinous muscle.

Technique To a depth of about 1 cun; perpendicular insertion.

BL

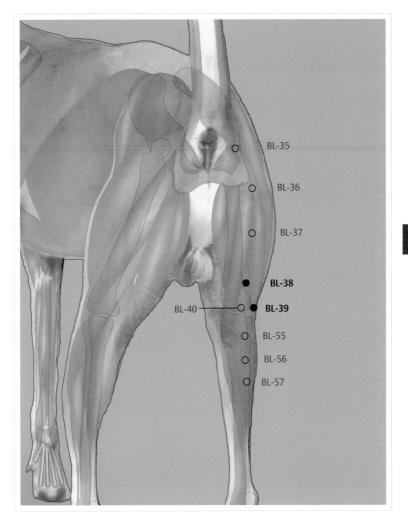

BL-35

BL-36

BL-37

BL-38

BL-40 —— **BL-39**

BL-55

BL-56

BL-57

BL

BL-40 Bend Center

委中 *Wei Zhong*

He-sea point, earth point, master point for the lower back and hip.

Effect Clears heat, eliminates summer heat, disperses dampness, cools the blood, removes channel obstructions, removes blood stasis, relaxes the tendons.

Indications Arthritis of the knee, hip, and in the lumbar area; all problems of the spinal column; weakness in the hind legs; caudal pareses and paralyses; gastrointestinal tract; genital tract; inflammatory skin disorders; fever; heat-related wasting; all problems of the urogenital system. Stabilizes and centralizes.

Localization In the middle of the popliteal fold, at the center of the transverse crevice in the popliteal fossa, between the biceps femoris and semitendinous muscle.

Technique To a depth of about 1.5 cun; perpendicular insertion.

BL

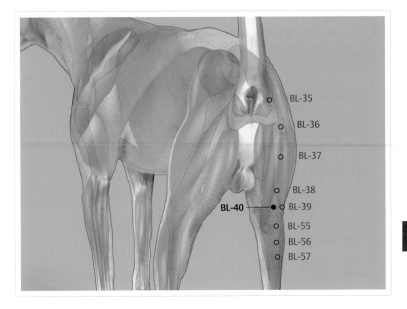

BL-35
BL-36
BL-37
BL-38
BL-40 — ● ○ BL-39
BL-55
BL-56
BL-57

BL

BL-41 to BL-54
These points form the external bladder channel. They have an effect comparable to the points on the inner bladder channel that lie roughly at the same level. As a result of the curve of the ribs, they are each associated with the point on the interior bladder channel that lies slightly more cranially. In isolated instances in the literature, they are therefore partly associated with one point further back on the interior bladder channel.

Localization   3 cun lateral to the dorsal midline and 1.5 cun lateral to BL-12 on the caudal edge of the spinous process of the second thoracic vertebra.

Technique   To a depth of about 0.5 cun; perpendicular insertion.

 Risk of pneumothorax.

BL-41   Attached Branch

BL

附分 *Fu Fen*

Intersecting point of the small intestine and bladder channels.

Effect   Especially effective for wind or trachea, eliminates wind-cold.

Indications   Pain and tension in the back of the neck, shoulder pain. Helps with the processing of losses.

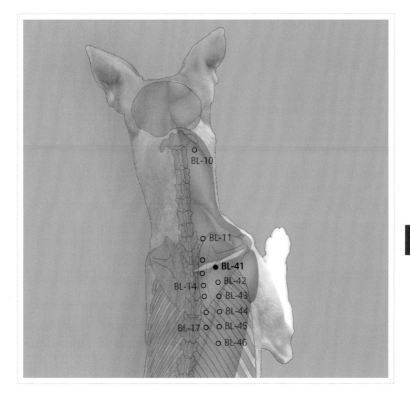

BL

BL-42 Corporeal Soul Door

魄户 *Po Hu*

Effect Houses the corporeal soul *po*, which is connected to the lung channel, and treats it for emotional problems, stimulates the lowering of lung *qi*, clears heat, regulates *qi*, checks coughing and asthma, activates the channel.

Indications Pain in the upper back as well as in the shoulders and in the area of the shoulder blades, stimulates the spirit, lung problems, pleuritis, vomiting. For the rejection of all instincts or for addictive behavior patterns. For the animal soul, stimulates the mind.

Localization 3 cun lateral to the dorsal midline and 1.5 cun lateral to BL-13 on the caudal edge of the spinous process of the third thoracic vertebra.

Technique To a depth of about 0.5 cun; perpendicular insertion.

 Risk of pneumothorax.

BL-43 *Gao Huang* Transport

膏肓俞 *Gao Huang Shu*

Effect Supplements *qi*, strengthens defense (*wei*) *qi*, nourishes the essence, nourishes lung *yin*, checks coughing and calms asthma, eliminates phlegm, clears heat.

Strong supplementing point for all three parts of the triple burner.

Indications All chronic diseases in weakened patients, chronic lung problems such as bronchitis, pleuritis. For a broken heart.

Localization 3 cun lateral to the dorsal midline and 1.5 cun lateral to BL-14 on the caudal edge of the spinous process of the fourth thoracic vertebra.

Technique To a depth of about 0.5 cun; perpendicular insertion.

 Risk of pneumothorax. Because of the potential effect on circulation, it is better to briefly apply moxa than to needle.

BL-44 Spirit Hall

神堂 *Shen Tang*

Effect Calms the disposition, moves *qi* along the channel, frees the thorax.

Indications Emotional problems related to the heart, respiratory problems, shoulder pain. Detachment due to shock or serious illness.

Localization 3 cun lateral to the dorsal midline and 1.5 cun lateral to BL-15 on the caudal edge of the spinous process of the fifth thoracic vertebra.

Technique To a depth of about 0.5 cun; perpendicular insertion.

 Risk of pneumothorax.

BL

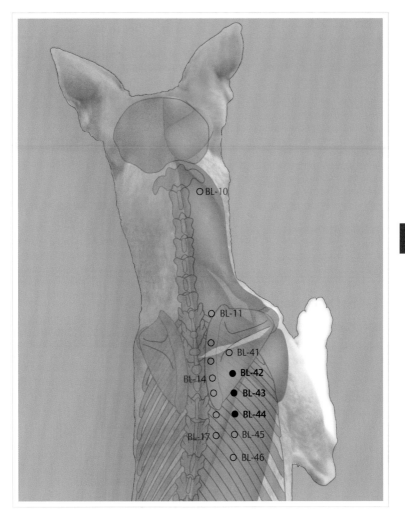

BL-45 *Yi Xi*

譩嘻 *Yi Xi*

Effect Eliminates wind, clears heat, lowers lung *qi*, relieves pain.

Indications Persistent back pain along the spine, lung problems, vomiting, states of exhaustion that do not want to end.

Localization 3 cun lateral to the dorsal midline and 1.5 cun lateral to BL-16 on the caudal edge of the spinous process of the sixth thoracic vertebra.

Technique To a depth of about 0.5 cun; perpendicular insertion.

 Risk of pneumothorax.

BL-46 Diaphragm Pass

膈关 *Ge Guan*

Effect Regulates the diaphragm, lowers rebellious *qi*, strengthens the center burner.

Indications Intercostal neuralgias, paravertebral pain, difficulty swallowing, dyspnea, urticaria.

Localization 3 cun lateral to the dorsal midline and 1.5 cun lateral to BL-17 on the caudal edge of the spinous process of the seventh thoracic vertebra, lateral to BL-17.

Technique To a depth of about 0.5 cun; perpendicular insertion.

 Risk of pneumothorax.

BL-47 Ethereal Soul Door

魂门 *Hun Men*

Effect Regulates and harmonizes liver *qi*, puts down roots to the ethereal soul.

Indications Emotional problems like frustration, anger, depression, related to the liver; regional muscle pain; pleurodynia; upper abdominal pain; distention, hepatopathies. Channels wild dreams.

Localization 3 cun lateral to the dorsal midline and 1.5 cun lateral to BL-18 on the caudal edge of the spinous process of the 10th thoracic vertebra.

Technique To a depth of about 0.5 cun; perpendicular insertion.

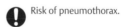 Risk of pneumothorax.

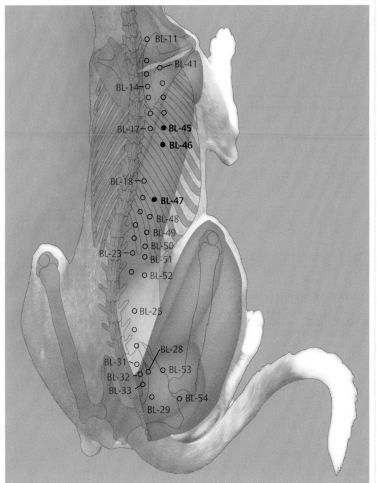

BL-48 *Yang* Headrope
阳纲 *Yang Gang*

Effect Regulates the gallbladder and clears damp-heat.

Indications Meteorism, hepatopathies, diarrhea or irregular bowel movements. Helps with decision-making.

Localization 3 cun lateral to the dorsal midline and 1.5 cun lateral to BL-19 on the caudal edge of the spinous process of the 11th thoracic vertebra.

Technique To a depth of about 0.5 cun; perpendicular insertion.

 Risk of pneumothorax.

BL-49 Mentation Abode
意舍 *Yi She*

Effect Supplements the spleen and stomach, regulates damp-heat.

Indications Treats the psychological aspect of the spleen, digestive disorders, hepatopathy.

Localization 3 cun lateral to the dorsal midline and 1.5 cun lateral to BL-20 on the caudal edge of the spinous process of the 12th thoracic vertebra.

Technique To a depth of about 0.5 cun; perpendicular insertion.

 Risk of pneumothorax.

BL-50 Stomach Granary
胃仓 *Wei Cang*

Effect Harmonizes the center burner.

Indications Digestive problems, constipation, colic, meteorism.

Localization 3 cun lateral to the dorsal midline and 1.5 cun lateral to BL-21 on the caudal edge of the spinous process of the 13th thoracic vertebra in the thoracolumbar transition.

Technique To a depth of about 0.5 cun; perpendicular insertion.

 Risk of pneumothorax.

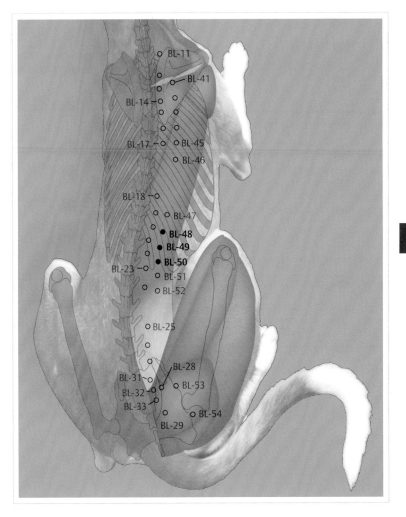

BL

BL-51 *Huang* Gate
肓门 *Huang Men*

Effect Regulates the triple burner, resolves stagnation, supports the mammae.

Indications Problems in the epigastrium, upper abdomen, hypochondrium, and spleen; mastitis.

Localization 3 cun lateral to the dorsal midline and 1.5 cun lateral to BL-22 on the caudal edge of the spinous process of the first lumbar vertebra.

Technique To a depth of about 0.5 cun; perpendicular insertion.

BL-52 Will Chamber
志室 *Zhi Shi*

Effect Like BL-23, but BL-52 even reinforces its effect, strengthens the spirit and will (*zhi*), supplements the kidney and essence, strengthens the lumbar region.

Indications Pain in the lumbar spine, nephropathies, inflammation in the genitals, impotence, urinary problems, difficulty swallowing, itching and oozing dermatitis.

Localization 3 cun lateral to the dorsal midline, on the external line of the bladder channel on the lateral edge of the longissimus muscle of the back, lateral to BL-23, on the caudal edge of the spinous process of the second lumbar vertebra.

Technique To a depth of about 0.5 cun; perpendicular insertion.

BL-53 Bladder *Huang*
胞肓 *Bao Huang*

Effect Opens the waterways in the lower burner, stimulates the transformation and elimination of fluids; while BL-51 works in the upper burner, BL-53 regulates in the lower burner, supports the penis.

Indications Urinary problems, cystitis, intestinal spasms, obstipation, diarrhea, problems of the iliosacral joint. Opens up the lower burner back after trauma.

Localization 3 cun lateral to the dorsal midline and 1.5 cun lateral to BL-27, at the end of the first third of the distance between the coxal tuber and the ischial tuber.

Technique To a depth of about 1 cun; perpendicular insertion.

BL

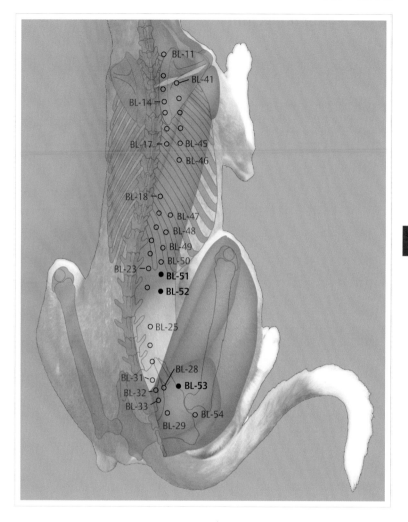

BL

BL-54 Sequential Limit

秩边 *Zhi Bian*

Effect Master point for the hind legs, supports the lumbar region.

Indications Pain in the hind leg, especially in the pelvis and hip; twisted pelvic joint; hip arthritis; myositis; ischialgia; dysuria; cystitis; prostate problems; diarrhea.

Localization Dorsal to the major trochanter at the end of the second third of an imaginary line between the coxal tuber and the ischial tuberosity.

Technique To a depth of about 1 cun; perpendicular insertion.

BL

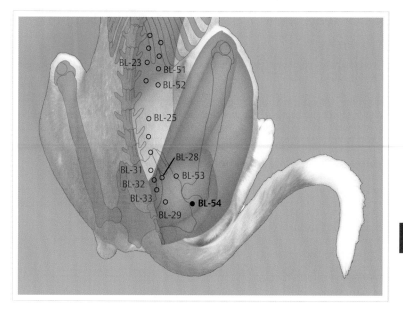

BL

BL-55 *Yang* Union

合阳 *He Yang*

Effect Activates *qi* along the channel, relieves pain.

Indications Swelling and pain in the posterior lower leg and lumbar region, pain in the genitals and due to hernias. Makes moving forward possible.

Localization Below BL-40 centrally in the gastrocnemius muscle at the level of the head of the fibula.

Technique To a depth of about 0.5 cun; perpendicular insertion.

BL-56 Sinew Support

承筋 *Cheng Jin*

Effect Moves *qi* along the channel, relaxes the tendons.

Indications Spasms and contractions in the distal hind legs and the lower spine, obstipation.

Localization Below BL-55 centrally in the gastrocnemius muscle.

Technique To a depth of about 0.5 cun; perpendicular insertion.

BL

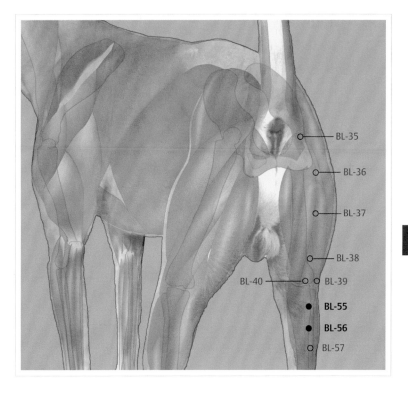

- BL-35
- BL-36
- BL-37
- BL-38
- BL-40 — BL-39
- **BL-55**
- **BL-56**
- BL-57

BL

BL-57 Mountain Support

承山 *Cheng Shan*

Effect Relaxes the tendons, strengthens the blood, clears heat, removes obstructions in the channel.

Indications Distal point for pain in the lower back, relaxes the muscles in the lower leg and paw, muscle spasms in the hind legs of racing dogs, problems with the Achilles tendon, blood in the stool that is caused by blood congestion, problems of the anus, prolapsed uterus and vulva, digestive problems, pain in the kidney region; for stabilization.

Localization On the transition from the gastrocnemius muscle to the Achilles tendon, centrally on the tibia.

Technique To a depth of about 0.4 cun; perpendicular insertion.

BL

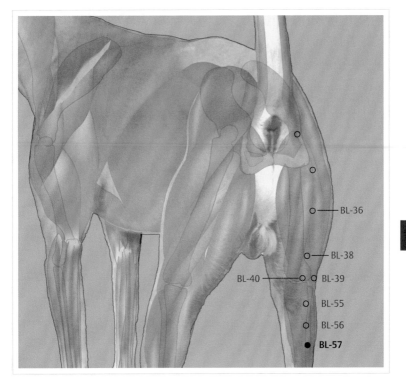

BL-36

BL-38

BL-40 —— BL-39

BL-55

BL-56

● **BL-57**

BL

BL-58 Taking Flight
飞扬 *Fei Yang*

Luo-network point.

Effect   Removes obstructions in the channel, expels wind from the small intestine and bladder channels, strengthens the kidney.

Indications   Hind leg debility, knee and ankle problems, nephropathies, cystitis. Relaxes in cases of excessive agitation and revitalizes in cases of immobility.

Localization   Lateral at the beginning of the Achilles tendon, caudal to the saphenous vein before it separates into the cranial and caudal branches.

Technique   To a depth of about 0.2 cun; perpendicular insertion.

BL-59 Instep *Yang*
跗阳 *Fu Yang*

Intersection point of the bladder channel and *yang* springing vessel (*yang qiao mai*), *xi*-cleft point of the *yang* springing vessel.

Effect   Strengthens the back, eliminates channel obstructions.

Indications   Hind leg debility, swelling in the ankle, pain and weakness in the lower back, discopathy. Discharges toxic emotions. In conjunction with LI-4 for physical poisoning.

Localization   Below the Achilles tendon, in front of the calcaneus, 3 cun above BL-60.

Technique   To a depth of about 0.2 cun; perpendicular insertion.

BL

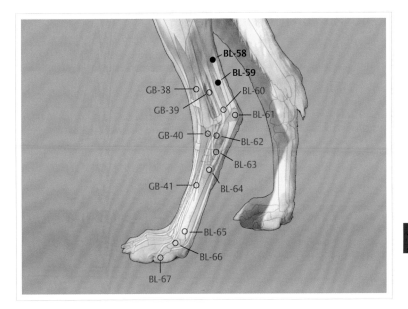

BL-60 Kunlun Mountains
昆仑 *Kun Lun*

Jing-river point, fire point.

Effect Eliminates wind and cold from the bones, clears heat, reduces *yang*, removes channel obstructions, relaxes tendons, strengthens the lower back and knees, relieves swelling and pain all over the body, promotes contractions during labor.

Indications Pain or disturbed sensibility in the ankle, back, head, and neck; cervical syndrome; ischialgia; paresis/paralysis of the hind legs; problems of the urogenital tract; obstetric complications; retained placenta; lymphadenopathy. Eliminates emotional coldness.

Localization Between the lateral malleolus and the calcaneal tuberosity, on a line with the tip of the malleolus between the bone and the Achilles tendon, exactly lateral to the centrally located point KI-3.

Technique To a depth of about 0.2 cun; perpendicular insertion.

 Contraindicated during pregnancy.

BL-61 Subservient Visitor
仆参 *Pu Can*

Intersection point of the bladder channel and *yang* springing vessel (*yang qiao mai*).

Effect Activates the channel and resolves obstructions there, relaxes the tendons.

Indications Weakness of the lower extremity, swelling and pain in the ankle, Achilles tendon problems, ischialgia, cervical syndrome. Removes the aftereffects of shock experiences when used in conjunction with GV-20, BL-11, and BL-23 as external dragon points, all used bilaterally.

Localization Lateral on the tip of the calcaneus.

Technique To a depth of about 0.2 cun; tangential insertion.

BL-62 Extending Vessel
申脉 *Shen Mai*

Opening point for the *yang* springing vessel (*yang qiao mai*).

Effect Eliminates internal wind, relaxes the tendons, strengthens the eyes, clears the spirit, removes obstructions in the channel.

Indications Swelling and pain in the ankle, back pain, neck pain, stagnation in the lateral back muscles, cervical syndrome, restlessness, insomnia (needle for sedation, supplementing in conjunction with KI-6), epileptiform seizures.

Localization In a depression just distal to the lateral malleolus.

Technique To a depth of about 0.2 cun; slightly oblique insertion from distal.

BL

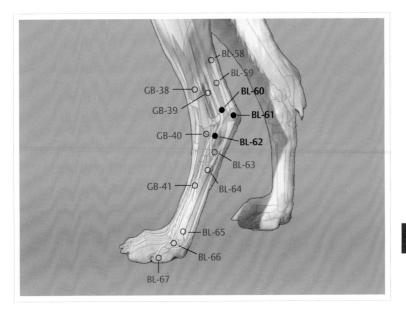

BL

BL-63 Metal Gate

金门 *Jin Men*

Xi-cleft point, intersection point with the *yang* linking vessel (*yang wei mai*).

Effect Eliminates wind, relaxes the tendons, relieves pain.

Indications Swelling, pain, and arthritis in the tarsal area, knee joint problems, epileptiform seizures, choppy movements.

Localization Below BL-62, distal to the calcaneal tuberosity.

Technique To a depth of about 0.2 cun; slightly oblique insertion from distal.

BL-64 Capital Bone

京骨 *Jing Gu*

Yuan-source point.

Effect Clears heat, eliminates wind, calms the spirit, clears the head and eyes, relaxes the tendons.

Indications Swelling, pain, and arthritis in the tarsal area; swelling and pain in the midfoot area; inflammations of the Achilles tendon; stiff neck; lumbago; burning pain during urination; cystitis; eye inflammations. Strengthens resilience of the back and psyche.

Localization Lateral to the base of the fifth metatarsal bone.

Technique To a depth of about 0.2 cun; oblique insertion from distal.

BL-65 Bundle Bone

束骨 *Shu Gu*

Shu-stream point, wood point, sedation point.

Effect Clears heat, reduces swelling, eliminates wind, clears the head and eyes.

Indications Tendinitis, sprains, swelling and arthritis in the ankle, hip pain, distal point for neck pain, kidney colic. When treated with moxa, it stimulates bone healing and breaks up rigid behavior patterns.

Localization Proximolateral to the head of the fifth metatarsal bone.

Technique To a depth of about 0.1 cun; perpendicular insertion.

BL

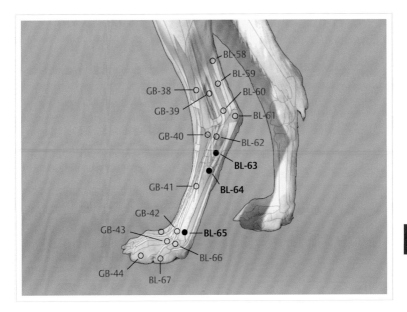

BL

BL-66 Foot Valley Passage

足通谷 *Zu Tong Gu*

Ying-brook point, water point.

Effect   Clears heat and the head, dispels wind.

Indications   Sprains and swelling in the ankle, tendinitis, cervical syndrome, acute cystitis, weakness of the anal sphincter. Strengthens in frightening situations.

Localization   In the depression in front of and below the metatarsophalangeal joint of the fifth toe of the hind paw.

Technique   To a depth of about 0.2 cun; perpendicular insertion.

BL-67 Reaching *Yin*

至阴 *Zhi Yin*

Jing-well point, metal point, supplementing point.

Effect   Dispels wind, clears the head and eyes, moves blood, eliminates obstructions along the channel.

Indications   Problems in the back, knee, ankle, and toe joints; incontinence and urinary retention; retentio secundinarum; eye inflammations; generalized itching; problems along the channel; fever.

Localization   On the lateral claw fold of the fifth toe of the hind paw.

Technique   To a depth of about 0.2 cun; oblique insertion from distal.

BL

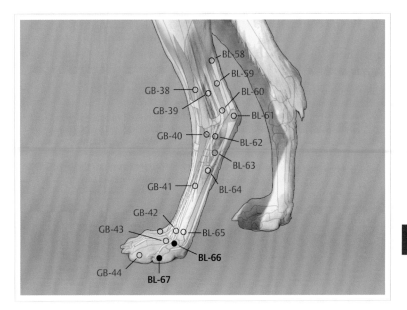

BL

18 Kidney Channel

Foot *Shao Yin* (*Zu Shao Yin Shen Mai* 足少阴肾脉)

External course: The kidney channel begins on the sole of the foot beneath the large paw pad. According to some sources, it begins on the medial side of the fifth toe of the hind paw. From there, it runs along the caudomedial aspect of the limb upward to the tarsus and across the knee to the groin. From here, the kidney channel runs 0.5 cun lateral to the midline, lateral to the controlling vessel (*ren mai*) to KI-21, lateral to the xiphoid process. Then it continues slightly more laterally on to KI-27.

Internal course: At the point KI-10 on the knee joint, a branch runs into the lower burner, connects with the bladder (*pang guang*) and kidney (*shen*), and then ascends to the lung (*fei*). From the lung, the channel continues on to the head where it connects with the eyes and ears.

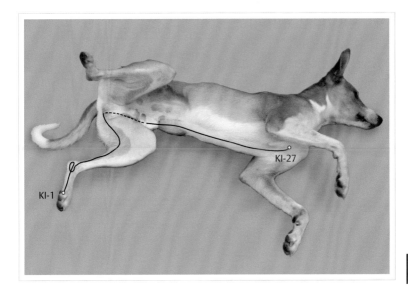

KI-27

KI-1

KI

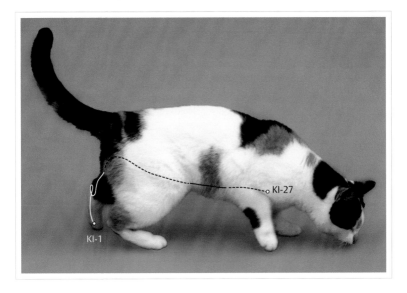

KI-27

KI-1

KI-1 Gushing Spring
涌泉 *Yong Quan*

Jing-well point, wood point, sedating point.

Effect Supplements *yin*, clears heat, suppresses wind, calms the spirit, restores consciousness.

Indications Shock; high fever; fear, in conjunction with high tension in the body or trauma; expecting catastrophes; distal point for all problems along the channel; functional disturbances in the kidney; epilepsy; paralyses; all forms of *yin* deficiency; localized problems; pain in the heel.

Localization Plantar between the second and third metatarsal bones, centrally underneath the large paw pad.

Technique To a depth of about 1 cun; oblique insertion from proximal to distal under the paw pad.

KI-2 Blazing Valley
然谷 *Ran Gu*

Ying-brook point, fire point.

Effect Clears deficiency of heat, regulates the kidneys and the lower burner.

Indications Arthritis of the ankle joint, sprained ankle, swelling, tendinitis, sexual dysfunction, vaginitis, scrotal pain, nephropathies, emotional immobility.

Localization On the caudomedial edge of the first metatarsal bone.

Technique To a depth of about 0.2 cun; oblique insertion upward.

KI-3 Great Ravine
太溪 *Tai Xi*

Shu-stream point, earth point, *yuan*-source point.

Effect Supplements the kidney and promotes essence, supplements kidney *yang*, supports the kidney function of fluid metabolism, strengthens the lower back and knees, clears deficiency of heat, regulates the uterus.

Indications Local point for the ankle joint; pain in the lower back; paralysis of the hind legs; growing pains; problems of the urogenital tract, especially the kidney; cystitis; functional disorders of the kidney; diabetes mellitus with weight loss; irregular estrous cycle; infertility. Helps to overcome fears through reflection.

Localization In a depression between the medial malleolus and the Achilles tendon at the height of the tip of the medial malleolus (opposite BL-60).

Technique To a depth of about 0.2 cun; perpendicular insertion or slightly oblique in a proximal direction.

KI

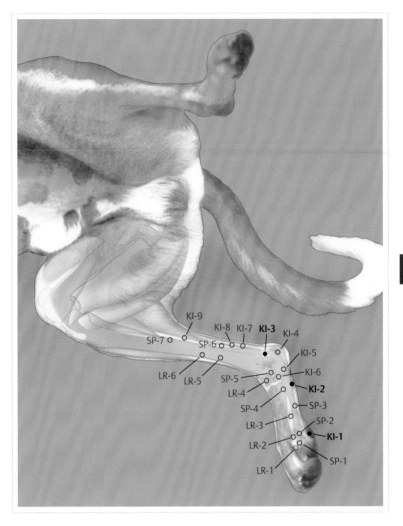

KI

KI-4 Large Goblet
大钟 *Da Zhong*

Luo-network point.

Effect This point is connected to the bladder channel, good for treating back pain that is due to chronic kidney deficiency.

Indications Arthritis in the ankle joint, pain in the lumbosacral area, dysuria, bladder problems, generalized sensation of cold, lack of energy. Resolves extreme hostility and distrust that lead to withdrawal.

Localization 0.5 cun caudodistal to KI-3 on the medial edge of the calcaneus at the beginning of the Achilles tendon.

Technique To a depth of about 0.2 cun; oblique insertion in a proximal direction.

KI-5 Water Spring
水泉 *Shui Quan*

Xi-cleft point, regulates the thoroughfare vessel (*chong mai*) and controlling vessel (*ren mai*).

Effect Stops acute abdominal pain, supports urination, promotes blood circulation, regulates the uterus.

Indications Acute cystitis, urethritis, urinary disorders including with gravel, pain and inflammation in the ankle. Strengthens the back against phobias.

Localization Caudomedial to the calcaneus at the transition to the head of the talus.

Technique To a depth of about 0.2 cun; oblique insertion in a proximal direction.

KI-6 Shining Sea
照海 *Zhao Hai*

Opening point of the *yin* springing vessel (*yin qiao mai*).

Effect Best point for nourishing kidney *yin*, causes the *yin* springing vessel (*yin qiao mai*) to bring *yin* energy to the eyes, cools the blood, supports the throat, promotes uterine function, calms the spirit, opens up the chest.

Indications Localized pain; skin disorders caused by heat in the blood; insomnia; epilepsy; uterine prolapse; irregular estrous cycle; thoracic pain; dry eyes and larynx, especially for older patients. For existential depression.

Localization In a depression distal to the medial malleolus of the tibia.

Technique To a depth of about 0.2 cun; oblique insertion toward proximal.

KI

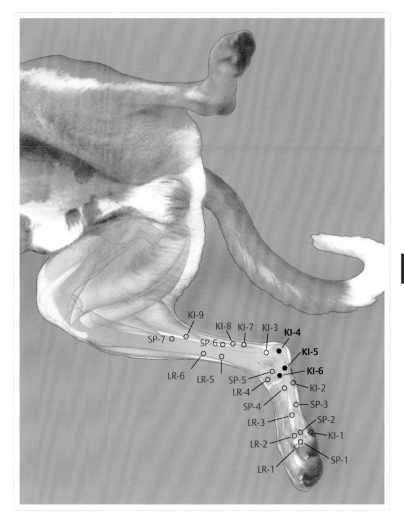

KI-7 Recover Flow
复溜 *Fu Liu*

Jing-river point, metal point, supplementing point.

Effect Supplements kidney *yang*, supports the kidney function of fluid metabolism, relieves dampness especially in the lower burner, regulates sweating, clears damp-heat, strengthens the lower back.

Indications Edemas, especially in the lower hind legs; pain in the lower back and ankle; problems of the urogenital tract, possibly with abdominal spasms; diarrhea; obstetric problems. Puts feelings in motion.

Localization 2 cun proximal to the tip of the medial malleolus, about 1 cun caudoventral to SP-6, on the cranial edge of the Achilles tendon.

Technique To a depth of about 0.2 cun; perpendicular insertion.

KI-8 Intersection Reach
交信 *Jiao Xin*

Xi-cleft point of the *yin* springing vessel (*yin qiao mai*).

Effect Clears heat, draws out dampness, stops abdominal pain, eliminates accumulations, regulates the controlling vessel (*ren mai*) and the thoroughfare vessel (*chong mai*) and hence also the estrous cycle.

Indications Spinal column problems, problems of the lower hind legs, orchitis, pain in the penis, dysuria, hernia pain, diarrhea, obstipation. Lacking sense of basic trust leads to excessive control and thereby to impotence.

Localization 0.5 cun further cranially at the level of KI-7 on the caudal edge of the tibia.

Technique To a depth of about 0.3 cun; perpendicular insertion.

KI-9 Guest House
筑宾 *Zhu Bin*

Effect Regulates *qi*, transforms phlegm, and clears heat.

Indications Muscle pain or spasms, painful hernias, abdominal spasms, for strengthening self-confidence.

Localization On the caudomedial edge in the middle of the length of the tibia.

Technique To a depth of about 0.8 cun; perpendicular insertion.

KI

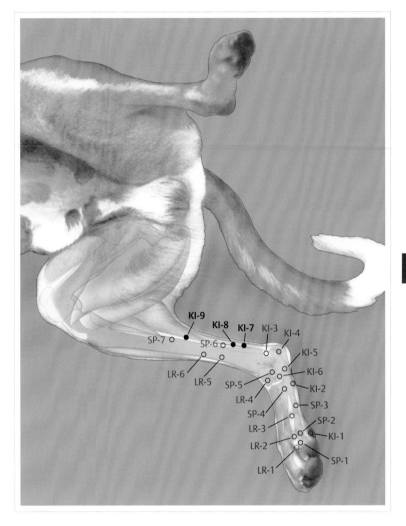

KI-10 *Yin* Valley

阴谷 *Yin Gu*

He-sea point, water point.

Effect Supplements kidney *yin*, expels damp-heat from the lower burner, moves *qi* along the course of the channel.

Indications Knee pain, fear-filled lethargy, urinary tract problems with painful or difficult urination, pain on the inner hind leg and in the knee joint, diseases of the genitals in male dogs and cats, prostatitis, vaginitis.

Localization On the medial side of the popliteal fossa, just cranial to BL-40 between the semimembranous and semitendinous muscles.

Technique To a depth of about 1 cun; perpendicular insertion.

KI-11 Transverse Bone

横骨 *Heng Gu*

Intersection point with the controlling vessel (*ren mai*).

Effect Regulates sexuality.

Indications Disturbed urination, incontinence, mastitis, pain in the genitals, impotence.

Localization On the cranial edge of the pelvic symphysis, about 0.5 cun lateral to CV-2.

Technique To a depth of about 0.5 cun; perpendicular insertion.

KI-12 Great Manifestation

大赫 *Da He*

Intersection point with the thoroughfare vessel (*chong mai*).

Effect Supplements the kidney, gathers essence.

Indications Urogenital diseases, impotence, infertility, uterine prolapse, mastitis, states of generalized weakness.

Localization 1 cun each cranial to KI-11 and lateral to CV-3.

Technique To a depth of about 0.5 cun; perpendicular insertion.

KI

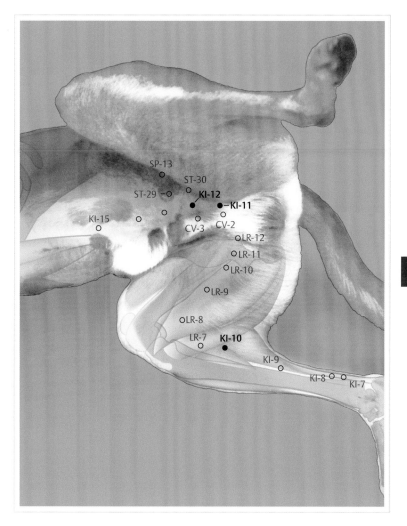

KI-13 *Qi* Point

气穴 *Qi Xue*

Intersection point with the thoroughfare vessel (*chong mai*).

Effect Regulates the lower burner.

Indications Urogenital disorders, mastitis, pain in the lower abdomen and genitals.

Localization 1 cun lateral to CV-4, 1 cun lateral to the midline halfway between the navel and the pelvic symphysis.

Technique To a depth of about 0.5 cun; perpendicular insertion.

KI-14 Fourfold Fullness

四满 *Si Man*

Intersection point with the thoroughfare vessel (*chong mai*).

Effect Moves *qi* along the channel, resolves blood stasis, supports the lower burner, regulates the waterways.

Indications Urinary incontinence, diarrhea, hernias, pain in the lower abdomen and genitals, postpartum problems.

Localization 2 cun caudal to the navel, 1 cun lateral to CV-5.

Technique To a depth of about 0.5 cun; perpendicular insertion.

KI-15 Central Flow

中注 *Zhong Zhu*

Intersection point with the thoroughfare vessel (*chong mai*).

Effect Regulates the lower burner and the intestines.

Indications Abdominal pain, especially in the lower abdomen; digestive problems; irregular estrous cycle; mastitis.

Localization 1 cun lateral to CV-7 and 1 cun from the midline.

Technique To a depth of about 0.5 cun; perpendicular insertion.

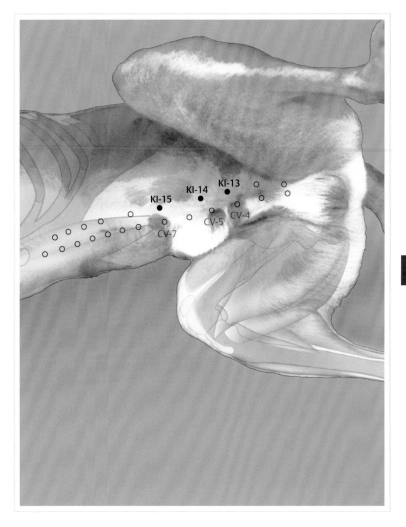

KI

KI-16 *Huang* Transport
肓俞 *Huang Shu*

Intersection point with the thoroughfare vessel (*chong mai*).

Effect   Moves *qi* along the channel, regulates and warms the intestines.

Indications   Digestive disorders, mastitis, sterility, pain in the lower abdomen and genitals.

Localization   1 cun lateral to CV-8 and 1 cun lateral to the midline next to the navel.

Technique   To a depth of about 0.5 cun; perpendicular insertion.

KI-17 *Shang* Bend
商曲 *Shang Qu*

Intersection point with the thoroughfare vessel (*chong mai*).

Effect   Moves *qi* along the course of the channel.

Indications   Colic, digestive problems, mastitis, pain in the upper abdomen. Releases trauma.

Localization   1 cun lateral to CV-10.

Technique   To a depth of about 0.3 cun; perpendicular insertion.

KI-18 Stone Pass
石关 *Shi Guan*

Intersection point with the thoroughfare vessel (*chong mai*).

Effect   Moves *qi* along the channel and resolves blood stasis, regulates the lower burner.

Indications   Digestive problems, mastitis, pain in the upper abdomen and stomach area, kidney stones. For petrified feelings.

Localization   1 cun lateral to CV-11 below the last costal arch.

Technique   To a depth of about 0.3 cun; perpendicular insertion.

 Risk of pneumothorax.

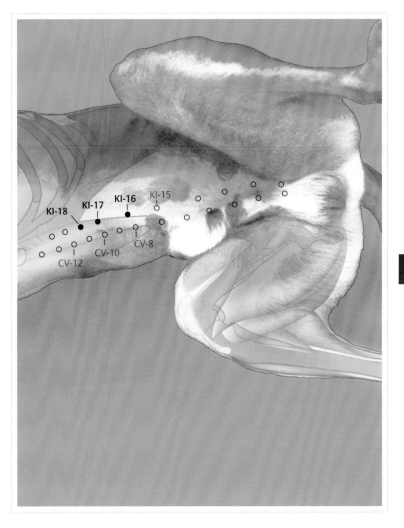

KI

KI-19 *Yin* Metropolis

阴都 *Yin Du*

Intersection point with the thoroughfare vessel (*chong mai*).

Effect   Lowers rebellious *qi*, harmonizes the stomach.

Indications   Weakened digestion in the stomach, upper abdominal pain with stagnation, mastitis.

Localization   1 cun lateral to CV-12.

Technique   To a depth of about 0.3 cun; perpendicular insertion.

 Risk of pneumothorax.

KI

KI-20 Open Valley

通谷 *Tong Gu*

Intersection point with the thoroughfare vessel (*chong mai*).

Effect   Harmonizes the center burner, transforms phlegm, frees the thorax.

Indications   Weakened digestion, upper abdominal pain, vomiting, mastitis. Connects with trust in the stream of life.

Localization   1 cun lateral to CV-13.

Technique   To a depth of about 0.3 cun; perpendicular insertion.

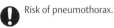 Risk of pneumothorax.

KI-21 Dark Gate

幽门 *You Men*

Intersection point with the thoroughfare vessel (*chong mai*).

Effect   Lowers rebellious *qi*, harmonizes the central and upper burner.

Indications   Colic; digestive problems; vomiting; mastitis; upper abdominal pain; feeling of congestion, also in the area of the thorax.

Localization   1 cun lateral to CV-14, caudolateral to the xiphoid process.

Technique   To a depth of about 0.3 cun; perpendicular insertion.

 Risk of pneumothorax.

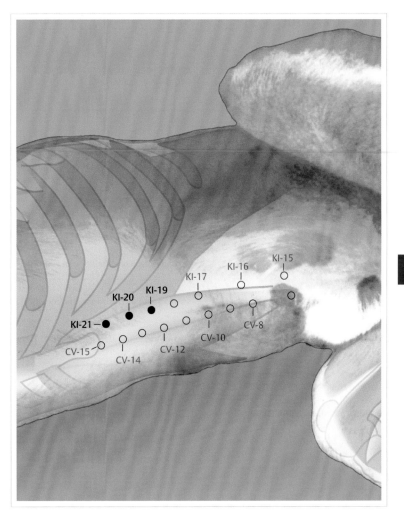

KI

KI-22 Corridor Walk

步廊 *Bu Lang*

Effect Frees the thorax, lowers rebellious stomach and lung *qi*.

Indications Bronchitis, pleuritis, dyspnea, mastitis in the upper area.

Localization In the fifth intercostal space, 1 cun lateral to the midline next to the sternum at the height of the elbow joint.

Technique To a depth of about 0.1 cun; perpendicular insertion.

 Risk of pneumothorax.

KI-23 Spirit Seal

神封 *Shen Feng*

Effect Frees the thorax, lowers rebellious stomach and lung *qi*, supports the upper teats.

Indications Intercostal neuralgia, pleurodynia, dyspnea, cough, mastitis of the upper teats, generalized weakness with vomiting. Stabilizes self-perception.

Localization In the fourth intercostal space 1 cun lateral to the midline and the sternum.

Technique To a depth of about 0.2 cun; perpendicular insertion.

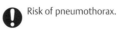 Risk of pneumothorax.

KI-24 Spirit Ruins

灵墟 *Ling Xu*

Effect Frees the thorax, lowers rebellious stomach and lung *qi*, supports the upper teats.

Indications Painful cough, intercostal neuralgia, lack of appetite with vomiting.

Localization In the third intercostal space, 1 cun lateral to the midline and the sternum.

Technique To a depth of about 0.2 cun; perpendicular insertion.

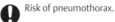 Risk of pneumothorax.

KI

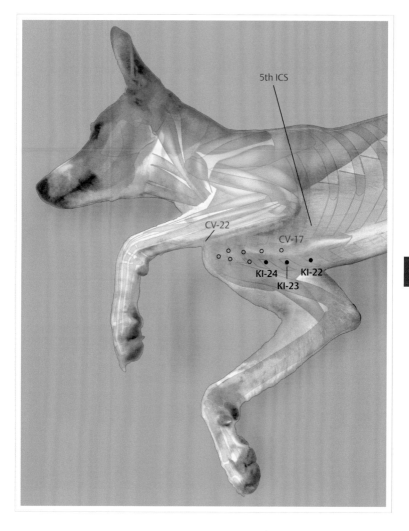

KI-25 Spirit Storehouse

神藏 *Shen Cang*

Effect Frees the thorax, lowers rebellious stomach and lung *qi*, supports the upper teats.

Indications Painful, spastic cough with shortness of breath, anorexia, esophageal spasms.

Localization In the second intercostal space, 1 cun lateral to the midline and the sternum.

Technique To a depth of about 0.2 cun; perpendicular insertion.

 Risk of pneumothorax.

KI

KI-26 Lively Center

彧中 *Yu Zhong*

Effect Transforms phlegm and lowers rebellious lung and stomach *qi*, frees the thorax, supports the teats.

Indications Painful, spastic cough with shortness of breath; cough with phlegm; pain in the thorax and flanks; mastitis in the upper teats. Strengthens self-confidence.

Localization In the first intercostal space, 1 cun lateral to the midline and the sternum.

Technique To a depth of about 0.2 cun; perpendicular insertion.

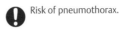 Risk of pneumothorax.

KI-27 Transport House

俞府 *Shu Fu*

Effect Frees the thorax, harmonizes the stomach, lowers rebellious *qi*, checks cough, calms asthma, dissolves phlegm.

Indications Spasmodic cough, asthma, bronchitis with profuse phlegm, chest pain, esophageal spasms. Enables conservation of the own reserves.

Localization Between the body and manubrium of the sternum and the first rib above the descending pectoral muscle.

Technique To a depth of about 0.2 cun; perpendicular insertion.

Pneumothorax and large vessels located underneath.

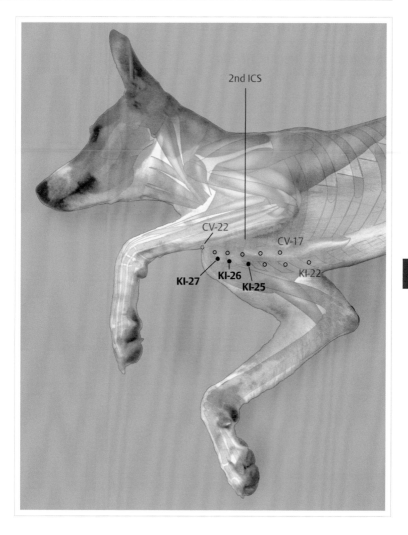

19 Pericardium Channel

Hand *Jue Yin* (*Shou Jue Yin Xin Bao Ma* 手厥阴心包脉)

The channel begins in the center of the chest and connects here to the pericardium. From there, a branch runs through the diaphragm downward into the three sections of the triple burner. Another branch runs from the chest to the beginning of the external course of the channel.

The external course of the pericardium channel starts in the fourth intercostal space lateral to the teat line, then continues along the inside of the forelimb to the elbow, and changes over to the palmar side, following the course of the median nerve. The end point is located, depending on the source, on the tip of the third toe of the forepaw medial to the claw fold.

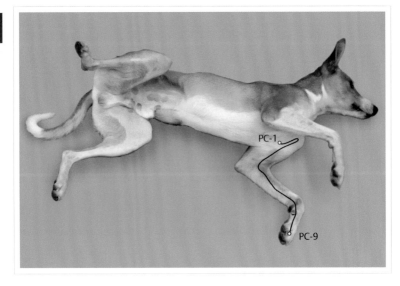

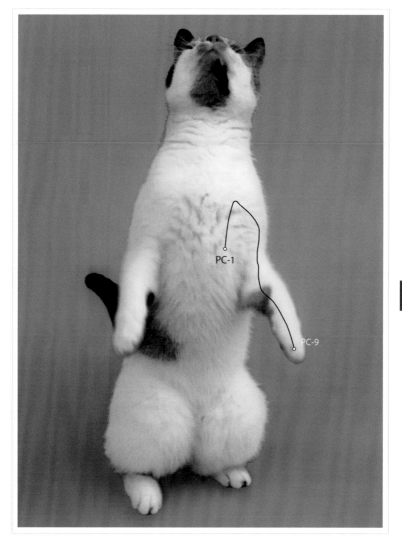

PC-1 Celestial Pool

天池 *Tian Chi*

Intersection point with the gallbladder and liver channels.

Effect Frees the thorax, transforms phlegm, regulates rebellious *qi*.

Indications Lymphadenopathy, especially in the armpit; cough; thorax pain due to cramping; neuralgia of the brachial plexus. Causes reopening after closing due to disappointment in the heart.

Localization In the armpit, between the fourth intercostal space and the medial aspect of the elbow, above the pectoral muscle.

Technique To a depth of about 0.3 cun; tangential insertion downward.

 Risk of pneumothorax.

PC-2 Celestial Spring

天泉 *Tian Quan*

Effect Frees the thorax, moves *qi* along the channel, strengthens the blood.

Indications Pain on the inside of the upper arm, shoulder, and thorax. Reconnects a warm heart, when sexual interests/duties have led to indifference.

Localization On the inside of the foreleg, directly below the shoulder joint.

Technique To a depth of about 0.5 cun; perpendicular insertion.

PC-3 Marsh at the Bend

曲泽 *Qu Ze*

He-sea point, water point.

Effect Cools and moves the blood, calms the stomach, calms the spirit, moves *qi* along the channel.

Indications Rashes, irritation, allergy and itching, gastrointestinal problems, heart problems, heat stroke, nervousness from too much closeness, explosive fits of rage, febrile spasms, pain in the elbow and forelegs.

Localization Roughly in the middle between LU-5 and HT-3, central in the elbow fold, medial to the tendon of the biceps muscle of the arm.

Technique To a depth of about 0.4 cun; perpendicular insertion.

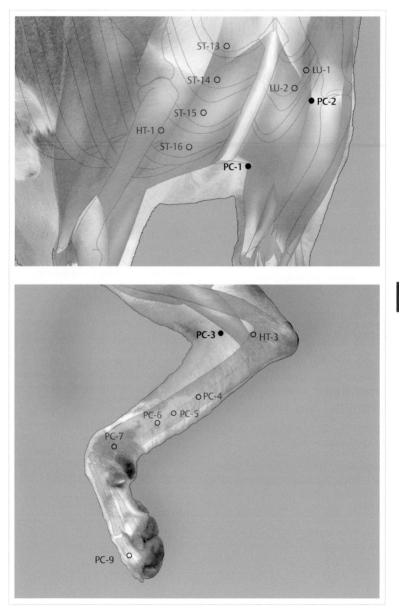

PC-4 Cleft Gate
郄门 *Xi Men*

Xi-cleft point.

Effect Cools the blood in the case of skin/haircoat problems.

Indications Heart and chest pain; tachycardia; anxiety; inappropriate fear among humans or animals, possibly after shock; mastopathy; reduced energy.

Localization In the middle of the lower foreleg, between the superficial flexor muscle of the flexor digitorum muscles and flexor carpi ulnaris muscles, 5 cun proximal to PC-7.

Technique To a depth of about 0.4 cun; perpendicular insertion.

PC-5 Intermediary Courier
间使 *Jian Shi*

Jing-river point, metal point, group *luo*-network point of the three *yin* channels of the forelegs.

Effect Transforms phlegm, calms the spirit, lowers rebellious *qi*.

Indications Elbow or arm pain, abdominal pain and vomiting, epilepsy, irritability, exaggerated hecticness after losing a partner.

Localization Medial in the middle of the forearm, at the start of the lower third, between the tendons of the flexor carpi radialis and superficial flexor muscles of the flexor digitorum muscles, 3 cun above PC-7.

Technique To a depth of about 0.3 cun; perpendicular insertion.

PC-6 Inner Pass
内关 *Nei Guan*

Luo-network point, opener of the *yin* linking vessel (*yin wei mai*).

Effect Master point for the chest and heart, strong point for calming the heart and spirit and for alleviating anxiety, regulates *qi* and blood, harmonizes the stomach.

Indications Inflammation of the carpal joint; heart problems; problems of the thorax; calms the spirit; problems in the upper abdomen; suppresses fear; promotes sleep; relieves travel sickness, nausea and vomiting; harmonizes stomach function; harmonizes inner sense of self with external activity.

Localization Medial 2 cun above the carpal fold, between the tendons of the superficial flexor muscles of the superficial flexor digitorum muscles and flexor carpi radialis muscles, lateral across from TB-5.

Technique To a depth of about 0.3 cun; perpendicular insertion.

PC

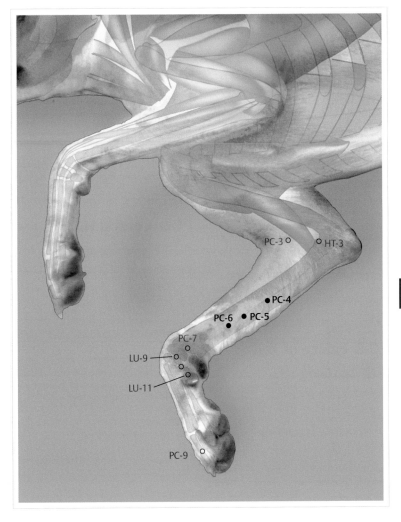

PC

PC-7 Great Mound
大陵 *Da Ling*

Shu-stream point, earth point, *yuan*-source point, sedation point.

Effect Good local point, calms the spirit, as strong as HT-7, clears heart heat, frees the thorax.

Indications Inflammation of the carpal joint, contractions in the paw and lower foreleg, heart and abdominal pain, poor circulation, epilepsy, irritability, pharyngitis, exaggerated sexual behavior, rashness, fluctuating emotions.

Localization Medial in the carpal joint fold, between the tendons of the flexor carpi radialis and flexor carpi ulnaris muscles, proximal to the radial carpal bone.

Technique To a depth of about 0.3 cun; perpendicular insertion.

PC-8 Palace of Toil
劳宫 *Lao Gong*

Ying-brook point, fire point.

Effect Clears heart heat, calms the spirit, harmonizes the stomach and clears the center burner.

Indications Tongue ulceration; gastritis; vomiting; pododermatitis; cardiac problems; epilepsy; mental disorders; pain in the lower foreleg, paw, and elbow; paralyses. Balances out fluctuating emotions and demanding hypersexuality.

Localization Between the third and fourth metacarpal bones, alternatively between the second and third metacarpal bones, proximal to the metacarpophalangeal joint, on the most proximal aspect of the central paw pad.

Technique To a depth of about 0.5 cun; oblique insertion from behind to the front and upward.

PC-9 Central Hub
中冲 *Zhong Chong*

Jing-well point, wood point, supplementing point.

Effect Eliminates heat, dispels wind.

Indications Resuscitation, shock point, heart disorders, pareses of the forelegs, allergies, fever. Emergency point for loss of consciousness from internal wind. In conjunction with TB-1, it promotes more caring behavior toward a partner.

Localization On the third toe of the forepaw medial to the claw fold.

Technique To a depth of about 0.2 cun; oblique insertion upward.

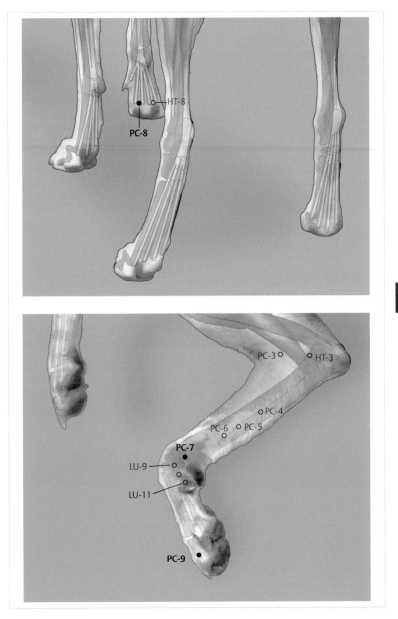

20 Triple Burner Channel

Hand *Shao Yang* (*Shou Shao Yang San Jiao Mai* 手少阳三焦脉)

The external course of the triple burner channel begins on the lateral side of the fourth claw and runs in a cranial direction to the carpus, where it changes over to the lateral side. From there, it runs in a caudal direction, up to the caudal aspect of the olecranon and shoulders, and then continues laterally along the neck via the throat.

After encircling the ear, the triple burner channel ends at the upper lateral edge of the orbit.

Starting at the shoulder, an internal branch runs to the pericardium and from there through the diaphragm into the three levels of the upper, center, and lower burner. A second branch runs behind the ear, and then through the ear toward the front, where it makes contact with the gallbladder channel.

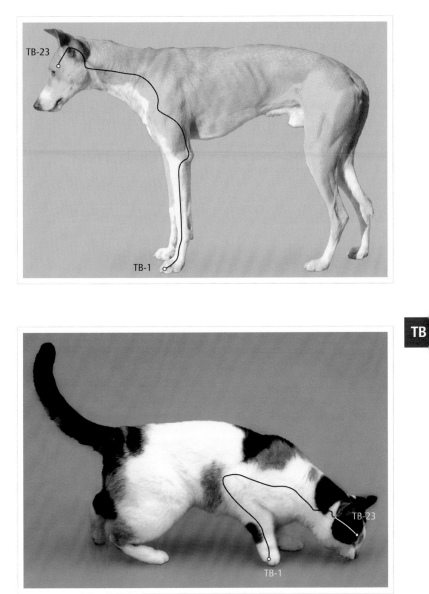

TB-23

TB-1

TB

TB-1

TB-23

TB-1 Passage Hub
关冲 *Guan Chong*

Jing-well point, metal point.

Effect Clears heat, dispels wind, moves blood, moves *qi* along the channel.

Indications Headache, laryngitis, otitis, hormonal dysfunctions, tendency to allergies, inflammations on the foreleg. Helps with appropriate social behavior that enables genuine interaction. Provides warmth and flexibility.

Localization Lateral on the fourth toe of the foreleg, 0.1 cun away from the claw fold.

Technique To a depth of about 0.1 cun; oblique insertion upward.

TB-2 Humor Gate
液门 *Ye Men*

Ying-brook point, water point.

Effect Clears heat, dispels wind, calms the spirit, supports the ears, moves *qi* along the channel.

Indications Otitis media, fever, laryngitis, gingivitis, inflammations of the claws and along the course of the channel, generally relaxing point. For enabling appropriate social behavior.

Localization Dorsally between the fourth and fifth toes of the foreleg at the level of the metacarpophalangeal joints.

Technique To a depth of about 0.2 cun; perpendicular insertion.

TB-3 Central Islet
中渚 *Zhong Zhu*

Shu-stream point, wood point, supplementing point.

Effect Clears exterior and interior heat, dispels wind, supports the ears, removes obstructions in the channel, regulates *qi*.

Indications Otitis; pain along the neck and forelegs; localized problems, such as periostitis or callus formation. For regulating extreme emotional instability with abdominal pain due to liver *qi* stagnation.

Localization Between the fourth and fifth metacarpal bones, in a depression proximal to the metacarpophalangeal joint, about 0.1 cun above TB-2.

Technique To a depth of about 0.2 cun; perpendicular insertion.

TB

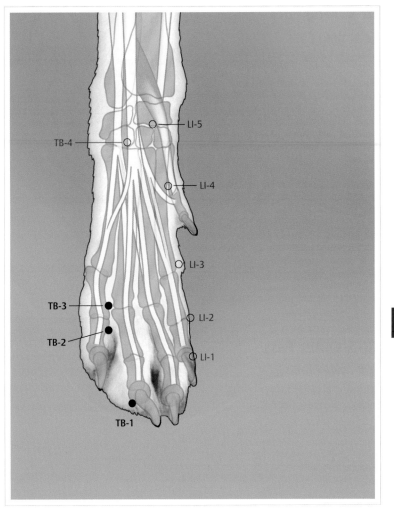

TB-4 *Yang* Pool
阳池 *Yang Chi*

Yuan-source point.

Effect Relaxes connective tissues and tendons, removes *qi* blockages in the channel, clears heat, regulates the stomach, promotes the transport of the fluids, supports source *qi*, supplements the thoroughfare vessel (*chong mai*) and controlling vessel (*ren mai*).

Indications Pain in the foreleg and shoulder, regulates and supplements the stomach function, pruritus vulvae.

Localization Dorsolateral on the carpus, in a depression between the radial and ulnar carpal bones, lateral to the tendon of the extensor digitorum communis.

Technique To a depth of about 0.2 cun; perpendicular insertion.

TB-5 Outer Pass
外关 *Wai Guan*

Luo-network point, opener of the *yang* linking vessel (*yang wei mai*).

Effect Opens up the exterior, dispels wind-heat, eliminates obstructions in the course of the channel, calms liver *yang*, supports the ears.

Indications Pain in the temporomandibular area, neck pain, pain in the forelegs, paralysis in the forelegs, ear problems, fever, headache, hormonal dysfunctions, prostatic hypertrophy. Opens the door appropriately for social contacts.

Localization Dorsal in the gap between the radius and ulna, near the radius, 2 cun above the carpus, across from PC-6.

Technique To a depth of about 0.5 cun; perpendicular insertion.

TB-6 Branch Ditch
支沟 *Zhi Gou*

Jing-river point, fire point.

Effect Clears heat, including blood heat; dispels wind; regulates *qi* in the triple burner.

Indications Pain in the foreleg, shoulder, lateral rib wall, and armpit; fever; obstipation; inflammatory skin affections, such as urticaria. Brings light and warmth into the psyche and regulates excessively demanding contact behavior.

Localization Between radius and ulna, 1 cun proximal to TB-5.

Technique To a depth of about 0.5 cun; perpendicular insertion.

TB

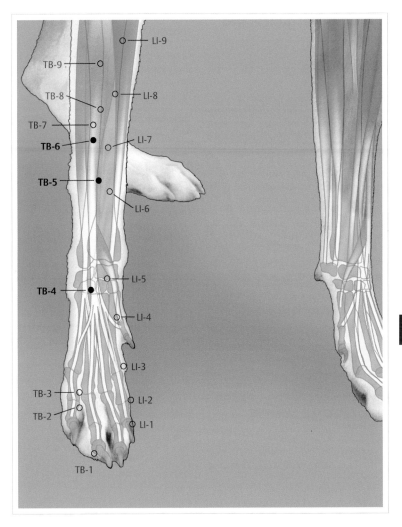

TB

TB-7 Convergence and Gathering

会宗 *Hui Zong*

Xi-cleft point.

Effect Eliminates obstructions in the channel; supports the eyes and ears; relieves pain in the eyes, temples, and eyebrows.

Indications Pain and spasms in the forelegs, epilepsy. To enable age-appropriate maturity.

Localization 0.2 cun lateral to TB-6 on the radial edge of the ulna.

Technique To a depth of about 0.3 cun; perpendicular insertion.

TB-8 Three *Yang* Connection

三阳络 *San Yang Luo*

Group *luo*-network point of the three *yang* channels of the foreleg.

Effect Clears heat, eliminates obstructions in the channel.

Indications Painful obstruction syndrome in the arm, neck, shoulder, back of the head as well as the lateral chest wall. Channels the energies forward.

Localization Laterally on the foreleg on the line between the transverse fold of the carpal joint and the lateral epicondyle of the humerus, 0.5 cun proximal to TB-6.

Technique To a depth of about 0.3 cun; perpendicular insertion.

TB-9 Four Rivers

四渎 *Si Du*

Effect Supports the neck and ears.

Indications Spasms and pain, paralysis of the forelegs, pain in the lower incisors, sudden numbness, sudden loss of voice. To prepare for new social contacts after disappointment.

Localization Ventral to the lateral tuberosity of the radius, centrally between the transverse fold of the carpal joint and the lateral epicondyle of the humerus, in the muscle channel between the extensor digitorum communis and extensor digitorum lateralis muscles.

Technique To a depth of about 0.5 cun; perpendicular insertion.

TB

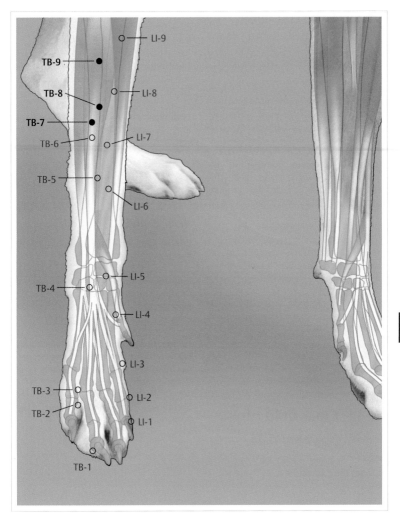

TB-10 Celestial Well
天井 *Tian Jing*

He-sea point, earth point, sedation point.

Effect Eliminates stagnations, relaxes tendons, calms the spirit, removes dampness and phlegm, resolves knots, regulates food (*gu*) *qi* and defense (*wei*) *qi*, clears heat.

Indications Removes swelling in the lymph nodes; swollen glands along the neck and throat; pain in the temporal region of the head, neck, and forelegs, especially the elbow; seizures; depression and mood swings; listlessness after psychological trauma; stress-related loss of appetite; inflammatory disorders of the respiratory tract. Stabilizes irascible or hysterical behavior and anchors the psyche.

Localization Centrally above the elbow, immediately proximal to the olecranon in the olecranon fossa.

Technique To a depth of about 0.5 cun; oblique insertion in a craniodistal direction toward the triceps tendon.

TB-11 Clear Cold Abyss
清冷渊 *Qing Leng Yuan*

Effect Eliminates heat and dampness, activates the channel.

Indications Pain in the lateral foreleg, especially in the withers and elbow. Provides warmth for social contacts.

Localization Centrally above the elbow and above the olecranon fossa, 1 cun above TB-10.

Technique To a depth of about 0.5 cun; in a craniodistal direction toward the triceps tendon.

TB-12 Dispersing Riverbed
消泺 *Xiao Luo*

Effect Eliminates obstructions in the channel.

Indications Cervical syndrome, pain, circulatory disorders and weakness in the forelegs, radial nerve paralysis. Replaces excessive control with zest for life.

Localization Central in the upper arm below the shoulder, in the groove between the long head and the lateral head of the triceps muscle of the arm.

Technique To a depth of about 1 cun; perpendicular insertion.

TB

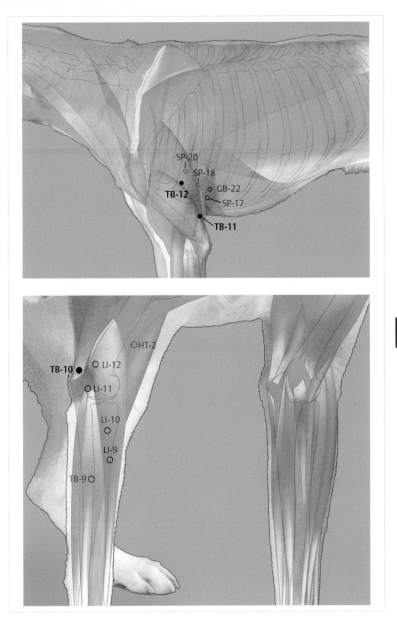

TB

TB-13 Upper Arm Intersection

臑会 *Nao Hui*

Connection point with the *yang* linking vessel (*yang wei mai*).

Effect Resolves obstructions in the channel, regulates *qi*, transforms phlegm.

Indications Pain in the foreleg and shoulder, swollen lymph nodes in the area of the neck.

Localization Lateral to the shoulder, directly at the caudal edge of the scapular part of the deltoid muscle, on the transition to the triceps muscle of the arm.

Technique To a depth of about 1 cun; perpendicular insertion.

TB-14 Shoulder Bone-Hole

肩髎 *Jian Liao*

Effect Clears heat, disperses wind and dampness, resolves obstructions in the channel.

Indications Localized shoulder problems, paralysis of the suprascapular muscle and radial nerve. Replaces excessive internal pressure and activity with joy.

Localization Caudodistal to the acromion, proximal to the greater tubercle of the humerus on the caudal edge of the deltoid muscle.

Technique To a depth of about 0.5 cun; perpendicular insertion.

TB-15 Celestial Bone-Hole

天髎 *Tian Liao*

Intersection point with the *yang* linking vessel (*yang wei mai*) and the gallbladder channel.

Effect Resolves obstructions in the course of the channel, regulates *qi* in the upper burner.

Indications Shoulder problems, neck pain and pain in the foreleg, chronic respiratory diseases. To cheer up when dejected.

Localization On the cranial edge of the trapezius muscle, at the height of the middle of the spine of the scapula, proximal to the acromion.

Technique To a depth of about 0.8 cun; perpendicular insertion.

TB

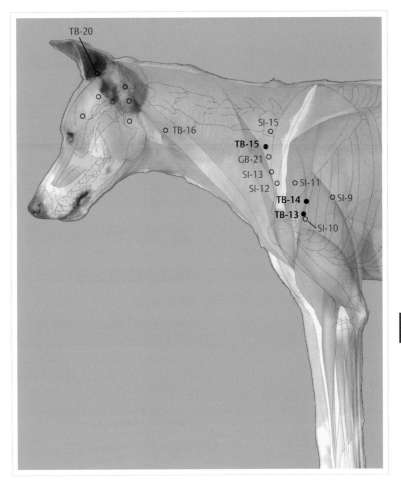

TB-20

TB-16

SI-15
TB-15
GB-21
SI-13
SI-12
SI-11
TB-14
SI-9
TB-13
SI-10

TB

TB-16 Celestial Window

天牖 *Tian You*

Effect Regulates and lowers the *qi*, supports the head.

Indications Neck pain, occipital neuralgia, torticollis. Helps to coordinate internal energies and balance them with cheerfulness.

Localization Cranial and ventral to SI-16 between the second and third cervical vertebrae.

Technique To a depth of about 0.5 cun; perpendicular insertion.

TB-17 Wind Screen

翳风 *Yi Feng*

Connection point with the gallbladder channel.

Effect Dispels wind, clears heat, supports the ears, resolves obstructions in the channel.

Indications Otitis, deafness, facial nerve paralysis, trigeminal neuralgia. Stabilizes in cases of excessive adaptation in social interactions.

Localization Ventral to the ear, in the depression between the mandible and mastoid process below the external acoustic opening.

Technique To a depth of about 0.3 cun; tangential insertion.

 Vicinity of the external carotid artery.

TB-18 Tugging Vessel

瘈脉 *Chi Mai*

Effect Calms wind, relieves fear, strengthens the ears.

Indications Facial nerve paresis, otitis, impaired hearing, impaired vision, epilepsy.

Localization Caudal to the base of the ear, in a depression between the external acoustic opening and the jugular process.

Technique To a depth of about 0.3 cun; tangential insertion.

 Vicinity of the external carotid artery.

TB-19 Skull Rest

颅息 *Lu Xi*

Effect Clears heat, calms fright, supports the ears.

Indications Facial nerve paresis, disturbed hearing, otitis, stiff neck. For excessive mental strain.

Localization Caudal to the auricle, at the height of the lateral canthus.

Technique To a depth of about 0.3 cun; perpendicular insertion.

TB

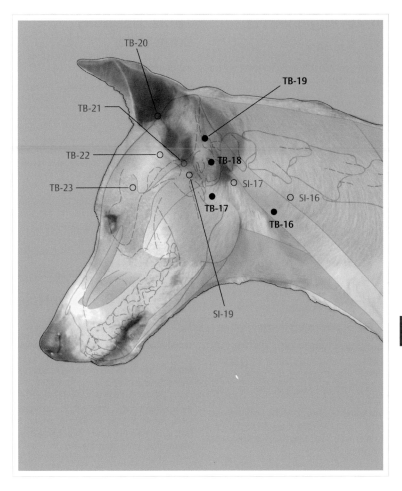

TB-20 Angle Vertex
角孙 *Jiao Sun*

Union point with the gallbladder and small intestine channels.

Effect Clears heat; supports the ears, teeth, and gums.

Indications Facial nerve paresis, otitis stiff neck, disturbed hearing, temporomandibular problems.

Localization On the dorsal attachment of the auricle to the temporal bone.

Technique To a depth of about 0.2 cun; perpendicular insertion.

TB–21 Ear Gate
耳门 *Er Men*

Effect Supports the ears, clears heat.

Indications Otitis, disturbed hearing, deafness, temporomandibular problems, gingivitis, toothache in the upper molars, disturbed equilibrium, trigeminal neuralgia.

Localization Above SI-19 behind the mandible, in the groove rostral to the edge of the tragus, rostral to the external acoustic opening.

Technique To a depth of about 0.5 cun; perpendicular insertion.

TB-22 Harmony Bone-Hole
和髎 *He Liao*

Union point with the gallbladder and small intestine channels.

Effect Eliminates wind and *qi* stagnation.

Indications Otitis, temporomandibular problems, disturbed hearing and equilibrium, facial nerve paresis.

Localization Caudal to the coronoid process of the mandible, dorsal to the zygomatic process of the temporal bone.

Technique To a depth of about 0.5 cun; perpendicular insertion.

TB-23 Silk Bamboo Hole
丝竹空 *Si Zhu Kong*

Union point with the gallbladder channel.

Effect Dispels wind, moves *qi* stagnation, clears the eyes.

Indications Eye problems, lipedemas, facial nerve paresis, headaches caused by liver *yang*, epilepsy. Enables harmony in living together through adaptation.

Localization Above the lateral corner of the eye at the height of the zygomatic process of the frontal bone.

Technique To a depth of about 0.3 cun; perpendicular insertion.

TB

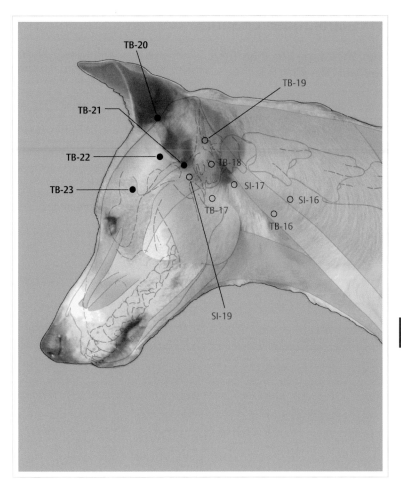

21 Gallbladder Channel

Foot *Shao Yang* (*Zu Shao Yang Dan Mai* 足少阳胆脉)

The gallbladder channel begins at the outer corner of the eye with a zigzag path across the head. Then it runs across the jaw joint and around the ear to the posterior base of the ear. From there, it ascends again across the forehead and then descends to the supraorbital foramen. It then runs caudally across the head to the dorsolateral aspect of the head and neck, across the shoulder and the lateral thorax, to the tip of the last rib. From here, it ascends to the height of the coxal tuber and the greater trochanter. Then it descends again along the lateral aspect of the hind leg down to the tarsus, where it changes over to the dorsolateral area of the foot. It ends on the lateral side of the fourth toe.

A branch of the gallbladder channel leaves the body's surface cranially by the lateral chest wall and runs from there deep into the body. Another branch runs to the gallbladder (*dan*) and the liver (*gan*). At the head, branches meet up with different points of the other *yang* channels.

GB

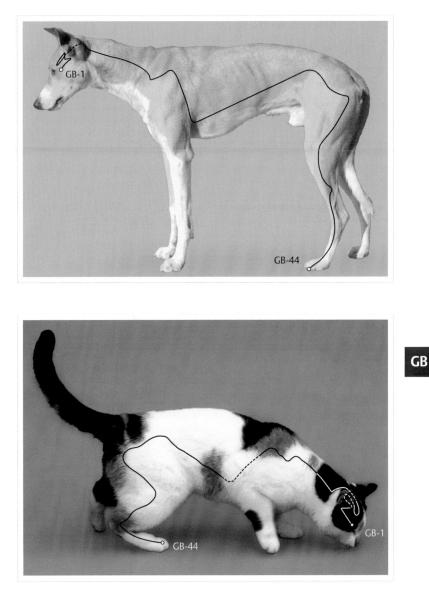

GB-1 Pupil Bone-Hole
瞳子髎 *Tong Zi Liao*

Intersection point with the small intestine and triple burner channels.

Effect Dissipates wind-heat, clears fire, brightens the eyes.

Indications Eye problems; facial nerve paresis; trigeminal neuralgia; important point for eye problems that are caused by liver fire, such as red painful eyes with iritis, keratitis, or conjunctivitis; blepharitis, also eyelid edema and cataract. Clears the vision and coordinates the visual angle also in a figurative sense.

Localization In a depression directly lateral to the outer corner of the eye and the orbit.

Technique To a depth of about 0.3 cun; oblique insertion toward the eye.

GB-2 Auditory Convergence
听会 *Ting Hui*

Effect Removes obstructions in the channel, clears external wind and heat, supports the ears.

Indications Local point for ear problems, for example, otitis media caused by external wind-heat; otitis externa; problems of the temporomandibular joint; gingivitis; facial nerve paresis. Opens up the ears again for advice from outside and for other perspectives.

Localization Below the anterior edge of the ear directly underneath SI-19, caudal to the condylar process of the mandible, in a depression that is formed when the mouth is open.

Technique To a depth of about 0.4 cun; perpendicular insertion.

GB-3 Upper Gate
上关 *Shang Guan*

Intersection point with the triple burner and stomach channels.

Effect Eliminates wind and supports the ears, resolves obstructions along the channel.

Indications Otitis, deafness, diseases of the teeth and jaw, facial nerve paresis. Helps to express bottled-up anger.

Localization With opened fangs in a depression on the upper edge of the zygomatic arch, halfway between the outer corner of the eye and TB-21.

Technique To a depth of about 0.3 cun; perpendicular insertion.

GB

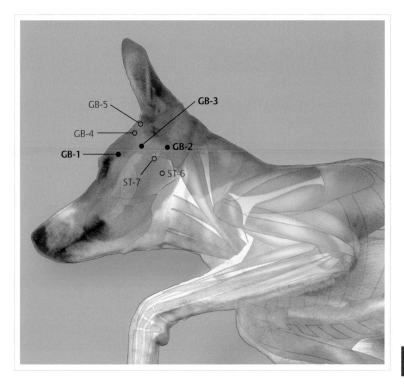

GB-4 Forehead Fullness

颔厌 *Han Yan*

Intersection point with the triple burner and stomach channels.

Effect   Eliminates wind and heat, resolves obstructions along the channel.

Indications   Otitis externa, facial nerve paresis, trigeminal neuralgia. Resolves doggedness and strengthens the ability for decision-making.

Localization   1.5 cun dorsal to GB-3, centrally located above the zygomatic arch.

Technique   To a depth of about 0.3 cun; perpendicular insertion.

GB-5 Suspended Skull

悬颅 *Xuan Lu*

Intersection point with the triple burner, large intestine, and stomach channels.

Effect   Eliminates wind and heat, resolves obstructions along the channel.

Indications   Otitis externa, facial nerve paresis, trigeminal neuralgia, continuous viscous nasal discharge. Clears blocked indecisiveness.

Localization   0.5 cun caudal to GB-4 between the middle and upper thirds of the line from GB-4 to GB-7.

Technique   To a depth of about 0.3 cun; perpendicular insertion.

GB

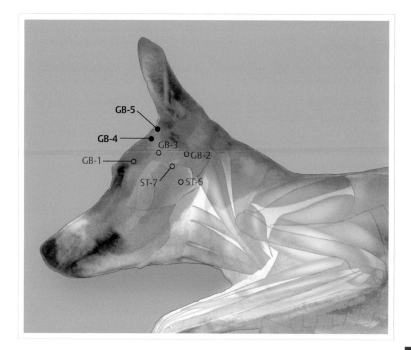

GB-6 Suspended Tuft

悬厘 *Xuan Li*

Intersection point with the triple burner, large intestine, and stomach channels.

Effect Dispels wind and clears heat, resolves obstructions in the channel.

Indications Headaches that are caused by liver *yang*, liver fire, or liver wind; conjunctivitis; swelling in the head; otitis.

Localization On the temporal bone, 0.5 cun caudal to GB-5, between the middle and upper thirds of the line from GB-4 to GB-7.

Technique To a depth of about 0.3 cun; perpendicular insertion.

GB

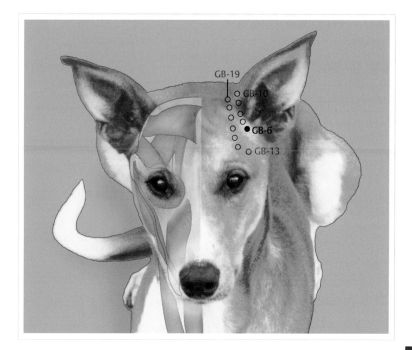

GB-7 Temporal Hairline Curve

曲鬢 *Qu Bin*

Intersection point with the bladder, small intestine, and triple burner channels.

Effect Resolves obstructions in the channel, supports the ear and head.

Indications Pain in the jaw joint and back of the neck, otitis externa.

Localization 0.5 cun caudal to GB-6 on the border of the anterior edge of the base of the ear.

Technique To a depth of about 0.3 cun; perpendicular insertion.

GB-8 Valley Lead

率谷 *Shuai Gu*

Intersection point with the bladder and small intestine channels.

Effect Eliminates wind, resolves obstructions in the channel, supports the head, harmonizes and resolves phlegm-cold in the diaphragm and stomach.

Indications Otitis, eye problems, pain in the frontal and lateral areas of the head. Has a collecting effect on absent-mindedness.

Localization On the temporal muscle medial to the attachment of the auricle, at the height of the ear canal directly dorsal to GB-7.

Technique To a depth of about 0.3 cun; perpendicular insertion.

GB-9 Celestial Hub

天冲 *Tian Chong*

Intersection point with the bladder and small intestine channels.

Effect Clears heat, calms the spirit.

Indications Otitis, gingivitis, eye problems, pain in the frontal and lateral area of the head, epilepsy, tendency to wind-related spasms.

Localization On the temporal muscle medial to the middle of the attachment of the auricle, about 1 cun dorsal to GB-8.

Technique To a depth of about 0.3 cun; perpendicular insertion.

GB

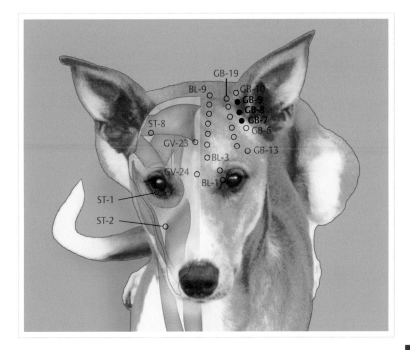

GB-10 Floating White

浮白 *Fu Bai*

Intersection point with the bladder and small intestine channels.

Effect Clears heat, supports the neck, activates the channel.

Indications Otitis, eye problems, pain in the frontal and lateral areas of the head, tonsillitis, struma, has an uplifting effect on the mood.

Localization Medial to the attachment of the auricle on a line about 0.5 cun dorsal to GB-9.

Technique To a depth of about 0.3 cun; perpendicular insertion.

GB

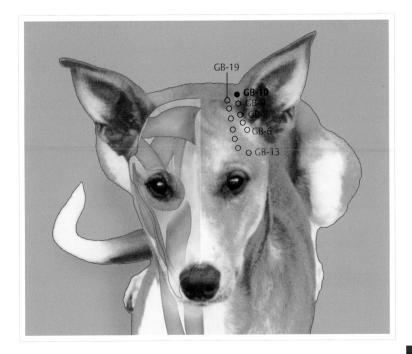

GB-11 Head Orifice *Yin*

头窍阴 *Tou Qiao Yin*

Intersection point with the bladder, small intestine, and triple burner channels.

Effect Activates the channel, clears the head, supports the sensory organs.

Indications Otitis, parotitis, eye diseases, tonsillitis, neck pain.

Localization On a line medial to the attachment of the auricle, in the middle between GB-10 and GB-12.

Technique To a depth of about 0.3 cun; perpendicular insertion.

GB-12 Completion Bone

完骨 *Wan Gu*

Effect Disperses wind, calms spasms, calms the spirit, supports the head.

Indications Parotitis, otitis, eye diseases, tonsillitis, neck pain. Channels rigidity that leads to impotent rage.

Localization In a depression posterior and inferior to the mastoid process, 1 cun caudal to GB-10.

Technique To a depth of about 0.3 cun; perpendicular insertion.

GB

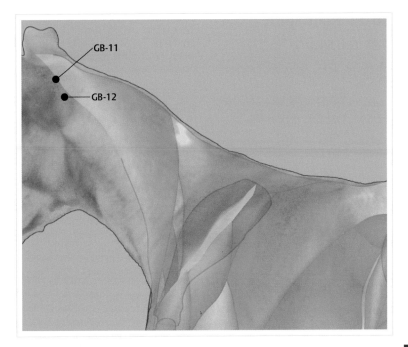

GB-13 Root Spirit

本神 *Ben Shen*

Intersection point with the *yang* linking vessel (*yang wei mai*).

Effect Calms the spirit, eliminates wind, clears the mind, removes phlegm.

Indications Eye diseases, facial nerve paresis, stiff neck, seizure disorders.

Localization 1 cun vertical above the outer corner of the eye.

Technique To a depth of about 0.2 cun; perpendicular insertion.

GB-14 *Yang* White

阳白 *Yang Bai*

Intersection point with the *yang* linking vessel (*yang wei mai*) and triple burner, stomach, and large intestine channels.

Effect Removes external and internal wind, supports the head, moves *qi* along the channel.

Indications Highly effective for expelling external and internal wind in the eye, facial paralysis, headaches, sinusitis, biliary colic. Also releases fixated thoughts.

Localization 1 cun above the center of the eyebrow, directly above the pupil in a depression in the upper edge of the eye socket, behind the zygomatic process of the frontal bone.

Technique To a depth of about 0.2 cun; oblique insertion toward the front.

GB-15 Head Overlooking Tears

头临泣 *Tou Lin Qi*

Intersection point with the *yang* linking vessel (*yang wei mai*) and bladder channel (*pang guang*).

Effect Removes wind, supports the head, moves *qi* along the channel.

Indications Eye diseases, tearing eyes in cases of wind, states of exhaustion with cold symptoms. For tendency to react by taking offense.

Localization Vertically above the pupil behind the zygomatic process of the frontal bone, at the beginning of the second fifth of a line between GB-14 and GB-19.

Technique To a depth of about 0.2 cun; oblique insertion toward the front.

GB

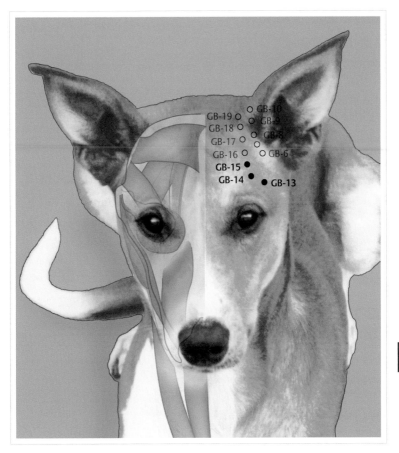

GB-19 ○   ○ GB-10
GB-18 ○   ○ GB-9
GB-17 ○   ○ GB-8
          ○
GB-16 ○   ○ GB-6
GB-15 ●
GB-14 ●   ● GB-13

GB

GB-16 Eye Window

目窗 *Mu Chuang*

Intersection point with the *yang* linking vessel (*yang wei mai*).

Effect Eliminates wind, clears the eyes, moves *qi* along the channel.

Indications Eye diseases, eyelid edema, vertigo. Promotes kindness and consideration, introspection, circumspection, and forbearance.

Localization Vertically above the pupil behind the zygomatic process of the frontal bone, at the beginning of the third fifth of a line between GB-14 and GB-19.

Technique To a depth of about 0.2 cun; perpendicular insertion.

GB-17 Upright Construction

正营 *Zheng Ying*

Intersection point with the *yang* linking vessel (*yang wei mai*).

Effect Supports the head, moves *qi* along the channel.

Indications Eye diseases, tooth problems, headaches. Stabilizes the personality, reduces fear.

Localization Vertically above the pupil at the height of the frontal edge of the base of the auricle, at the beginning of the fourth fifth of the line between GB-14 and GB-19.

Technique To a depth of about 0.3 cun; perpendicular insertion.

GB-18 Spirit Support

承灵 *Cheng Ling*

Intersection point with the *yang* springing vessel (*yang qiao mai*).

Effect Supports the head, moves *qi* along the channel, lowers lung *qi*.

Indications Eye diseases, rhinitis, stiff neck.

Localization Vertically above the pupil in the center of the attachment of the auricle, at the beginning of the last fifths of the line between GB-14 and GB-19.

Technique To a depth of about 0.3 cun; perpendicular insertion.

GB

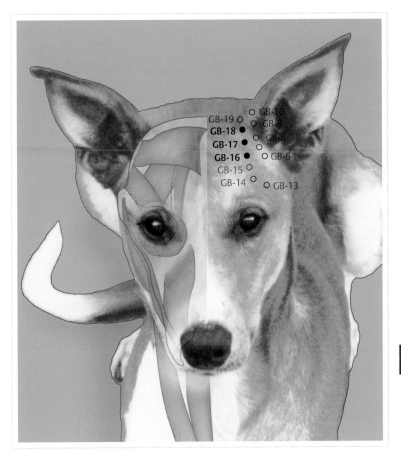

GB-19 Brain Hollow

脑空 *Nao Kong*

Intersection point with the *yang* linking vessel (*yang wei mai*).

Effect Draws out wind, clears the sensory organs, supports the head, resolves *qi* blockages along the channel.

Indications Neck pain, nosebleeds, photophobia, sinusitis, epilepsy, fearfulness, tense shoulders and neck.

Localization Lateral on the nuchal crest on a continuation of the line between GB-14 and GB-18.

Technique To a depth of about 0.2 cun; oblique insertion toward the front and upward.

GB

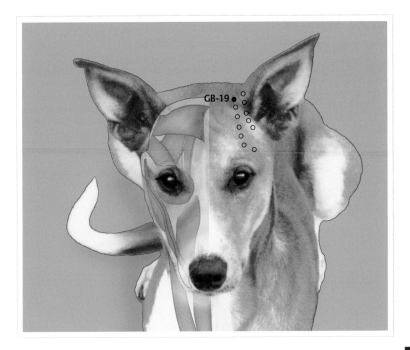

GB-20 Wind Pool

风池 *Feng Chi*

Intersection point with the *yang* springing vessel (*yang qiao mai*), *yang* linking vessel (*yang wei mai*), and triple burner channel.

Effect Disperses external wind-heat and wind-cold, disperses internal wind, clears the sensory organs, activates the channel, supports the head, clears the mind.

Indications Problems of the ears, eyes, and neck; epilepsy; fever; influenza; torticollis; circulatory disorders in the brain; spasms; pharyngitis; rhinitis; problems in the hip joints.

Localization Rostromedial to the lateral mass of the atlas, caudomedial to the jugular process of the occiput, at the height of the base of the ear, between the bellies of the sternomastoid and sterno-occipital muscles, lateral to GV-16.

Technique To a depth of about 0.8 cun; oblique insertion from the back in the direction of the contralateral eye.

GB

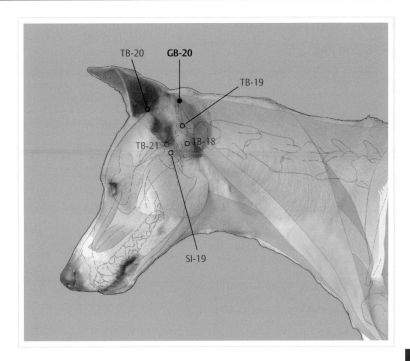

TB-20

GB-20

TB-19

TB-21

TB-18

SI-19

GB

GB-21 Shoulder Well

肩井 *Jian Jing*

Intersection point with the *yang* linking vessel (*yang wei mai*) and the triple burner and stomach channels.

Effect Regulates *qi*, strongly lowering; activates the channel; transforms and reduces phlegm; eliminates knots; promotes lactation; accelerates delivery, is therefore contraindicated during pregnancy.

Indications Local point for treating painful blockages in the shoulder and neck region; struma; empirical point for all types of gynecological problems, such as retained placenta; postpartum bleeding; mastitis; lactation problems.

Localization In the middle of the neck in front of the shoulder blade, midway between GV-14 and the acromion, between the sixth and seventh cervical vertebrae.

Technique To a depth of about 1 cun; perpendicular insertion.

 Contraindicated during pregnancy.

GB-22 Armpit Abyss

渊腋 *Yuan Ye*

Effect Regulates *qi*, frees the thorax, supports the axilla.

Indications Intercostal neuralgias, rib blockages, pleuritis, axillary lymphadenitis, shoulder pain.

Localization In the fifth intercostal space between the latissimus dorsi and pectoralis profundus muscles in the armpit.

Technique To a depth of about 0.3 cun; tangential insertion.

 Risk of pneumothorax.

GB-23 Sinew Seat

辄筋 *Zhe Jin*

Intersection point with the bladder channel.

Effect Regulates *qi* in the triple burner, frees the thorax, lowers rebellious *qi*. Frees the *shen*.

Indications Upper abdominal pain, difficulty breathing, functional heart problems, cholecystopathies. Has a flash-like brightening effect.

Localization In the sixth intercostal space, about 1 cun below SP-21 on the pectoral muscle.

Technique To a depth of about 0.3 cun; tangential insertion.

 Risk of pneumothorax.

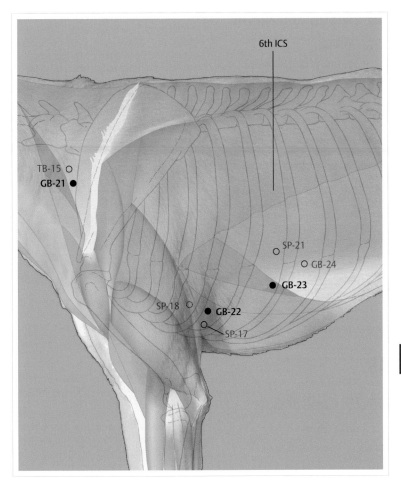

6th ICS

TB-15 ○
GB-21 ●

SP-21 ○
○ GB-24
● **GB-23**

SP-18 ○
● **GB-22**
○
SP-17

GB

GB-24 Sun and Moon
日月 *Ri Yue*

Mu-alarm point of the gallbladder.

Effect   Resolves damp-heat, supports the functions of the gallbladder (*dan*) and liver (*gan*), soothes liver *qi*.

Indications   Damp-heat in the gallbladder (*dan*) and liver (*gan*), such as icterus; hypochondriac pain; biliary stones; feeling of heaviness; listlessness; nausea; sticky yellow tongue coating; difficulty breathing.

Localization   In the seventh intercostal space at the level of the costochondral junction, corresponds to the sixth intercostal space from behind (there are, however, also references in the literature to the 10th intercostal space, which corresponds to the third one from behind).

Technique   To a depth of about 0.3 cun; tangential insertion.

 Risk of pneumothorax.

GB-25 Capital Gate
京门 *Jing Men*

Mu-alarm point of the kidneys.

Effect   Supplements the spleen and kidneys, regulates water flow, strengthens the lumbar area.

Indications   Pain in the lumbar area, intercostal neuralgia, kidney disorders, infertility, biliary colic, mastitis. Reduces emotional fluctuations, balances decision-making processes in leadership situations.

Localization   On the caudal edge of the free end of the 13th rib.

Technique   To a depth of about 0.3 cun; tangential insertion.

 Risk of pneumothorax.

GB-26 Girdling Vessel
带脉 *Dai Mai*

Intersection point with the girdling vessel (*dai mai*).

Effect   Resolves damp-heat, regulates the uterus, regulates the girdling vessel, activates the channel.

Indications   Endometritis, abdominal pain, diagnostically useful for congestion in the girdling vessel, inflammatory disorders in the urogenital area. Regulates internal tension and thirst for action.

Localization   2 cun below the external bladder channel, cranial to the foremost edge of the coxal tuber.

Technique   To a depth of about 0.5 cun; perpendicular insertion.

GB

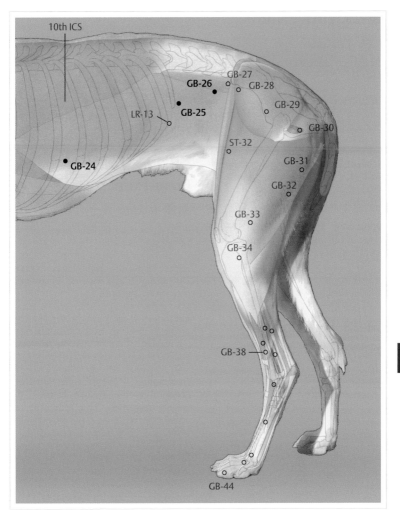

GB-27 Fifth Pivot
五枢 *Wu Shu*

Intersection point with the girdling vessel (*dai mai*).

Effect Regulates the girdling vessel (*dai mai*) and the lower burner, transforms stagnation.

Indications Diagnostic point for hip problems, treats all problems of the posterior back, painful defecation, uterine prolapse, pain in the testicles and lower abdomen.

Localization Directly in front of the lower corner of the ilium, on the anterior superior iliac spine.

Technique To a depth of about 0.5 cun; perpendicular insertion.

GB-28 Linking Path
维道 *Wei Dao*

Intersection point with the girdling vessel (*dai mai*).

Effect Regulates the girdling vessel (*dai mai*) and the lower burner, transforms stagnation.

Indications Hip pain, endometritis, chronic constipation, pain in the lower burner, orchitis, sterility.

Localization Below the ilium, about 0.5 cun caudal to GB-27, at the beginning of the spine of the ala.

Technique To a depth of about 0.5 cun; perpendicular insertion.

GB-29 Squatting Bone-Hole
居髎 *Ju Liao*

Intersection point with the *yang* springing vessel (*yang qiao mai*).

Effect Eliminates wind-damp, resolves obstructions in the channel, supports the hind leg and hip area.

Indications Local point for all painful hip problems, for pain in the back and hind leg, paralysis of the hind leg, shoulder pain, orchitis, endometritis, cystitis.

Localization In front of the hip joint, one-third of the distance between the greater trochanter of the femur and the dorsal edge of the posterior superior iliac spine.

Technique To a depth of about 2 cun; perpendicular insertion.

GB

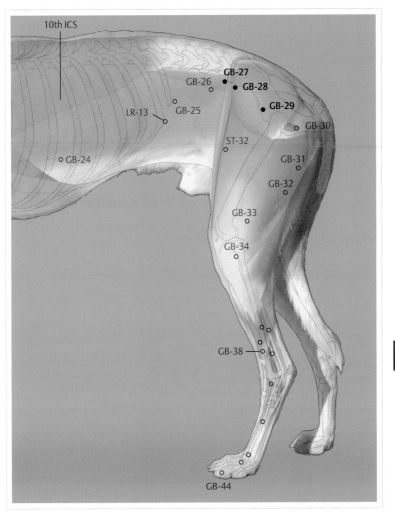

10th ICS

GB-27
GB-26
GB-28
GB-25
GB-29
LR-13
GB-30
ST-32
GB-24
GB-31
GB-32
GB-33
GB-34
GB-38
GB-44

GB

GB-30 Jumping Round

环跳 *Huan Tiao*

Effect Intersection point with the bladder channel.

Removes obstructions in the channel, supplements *qi* and blood, resolves damp-heat.

Indications Sciatica with pain that stretches across the lateral side of the leg, paralysis of the hind leg, hip joint dysplasia, hemiplegia. Frees from a perceived lack of freedom and constriction.

Localization Caudal to the greater trochanter of the femur, halfway between the trochanter and the ischial tuberosity.

In classic veterinary acupuncture, *huan tiao* is described as located directly in front of the greater trochanter; the localization of GB-30 is referred to as *huan hou*.

Technique To a depth of about 2 cun; perpendicular insertion.

GB

GB-31 Wind Market

风市 *Feng Shi*

Effect Expels wind, relaxes the tendons, strengthens the hind legs, relieves itching.

Indications Itching all over the body, paralysis of the hind legs, pain and swelling in the hind legs and lower back, hip joint problems, ischialgia.

Localization On the posterior edge and approximately in the middle of the thigh, between the biceps muscle of the thigh and the semitendinous muscle, 7 cun above the knee fold.

Technique To a depth of about 1 cun; perpendicular insertion.

GB-32 Central River

中渎 *Zhong Du*

Effect Expels wind and cold-damp.

Indications Paralysis, swelling or weakness in the hind legs, pain in the hind legs and lower back, hip joint problems, ischialgia.

Localization On the posterior edge and approximately in the middle of the thigh, between the biceps muscle of the thigh and the semitendinous muscle, 5 cun above the knee fold.

Technique To a depth of about 1 cun; perpendicular insertion.

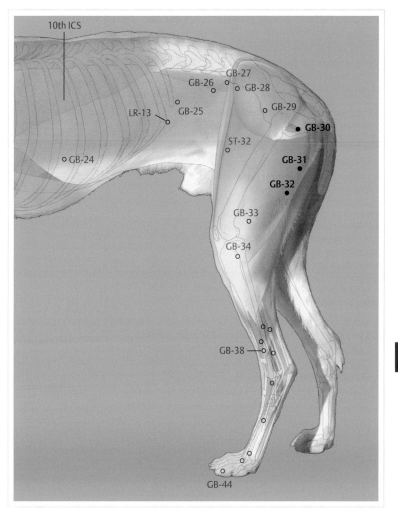

GB

GB-33 Knee *Yang* Joint

膝阳关 *Xi Yang Guan*

Effect Relaxes the tendons, supports the joints, cold *bi* (impediment) syndrome in the lateral knee, eliminates wind-damp.

Indications Particularly contractions of the lateral aspects of the ligaments and tendons in this area, wind *bi* (impediment) syndrome in the knee with a feeling of numbness, reduced mobility and swelling in the knee joint. Facilitates appropriate adaptation to external conditions.

Localization In a depression proximal to the lateral epicondyle of the femur at the knee, between the tendon of the biceps muscle of the thigh and the femur, 3 cun above GB-34 when the knee is bent.

Technique To a depth of about 1 cun; perpendicular insertion.

GB-34 *Yang* Mound Spring

阳陵泉 *Yang Ling Quan*

He-sea point, earth point, *hui*-meeting point for the tendons.

Effect Removes channel obstructions, resolves damp heat in gallbladder (*dan*) and liver (*gan*), supports the smooth flow of liver *qi* through the whole body, calms rebellious *qi*, relaxes the tendons, harmonizes *shao yang*.

Indications Important point for improving the flow of *qi* and blood in the legs, especially in the knee; knee joint problems; atrophied muscles; muscle contractions and spasms; tendon pathologies; pain in the lateral rib area. Can accompany manifested anger.

Localization Inferolateral to the knee, in a depression cranial and distal to the head of the fibula.

Technique To a depth of about 1 cun; perpendicular insertion.

GB

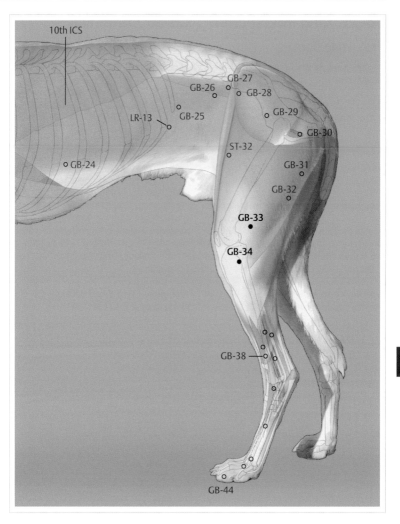

10th ICS

GB-27
GB-26
GB-28
GB-25
LR-13
GB-29
GB-30
ST-32
GB-24
GB-31
GB-32
GB-33
GB-34
GB-38
GB-44

GB-35 *Yang* Intersection

阳交 *Yang Jiao*

Xi-cleft point of the *yang* linking vessel (*yang wei mai*).

Effect Removes channel congestion, relaxes tendons and nerves, stops pain.

Indications Pain along the gallbladder channel that is accompanied by stiffness, numbness, and spasms in the leg muscles; asthmatic bronchitis with states of fear.

Localization In the middle of the posterior edge of the fibula, halfway between the lateral malleolus and the head of the fibula, at the same height on a slightly oblique line as GB-36 and BL-58 caudally and ST-40 and ST-39 cranially.

Technique To a depth of about 0.5 cun; perpendicular insertion.

GB-36 Outer Hill

外丘 *Wai Qiu*

Xi-cleft point.

Effect Eliminates channel obstructions, clears pathogenic heat, eliminates channel congestion, stops pain.

Indications Indicated for all cases of acute pain on the channel or in the organ, especially in the lower leg and lateral neck area. Increases levelheadedness in cases with tendency to irascibility.

Localization Halfway between the lateral malleolus and the head of the fibula, at the same height on a slightly oblique line as BL-58 caudally, and GB-35, ST-40, and ST-39 cranially.

Technique To a depth of about 0.5 cun; perpendicular insertion.

GB

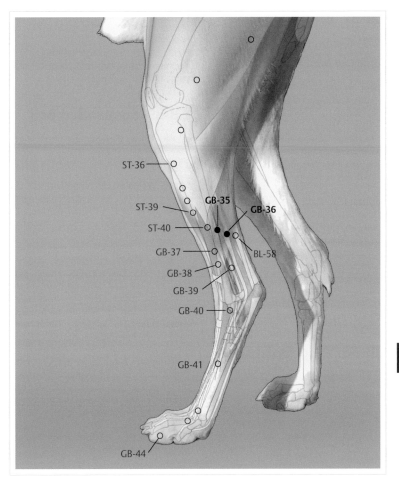

ST-36

ST-39

ST-40

GB-35

GB-36

BL-58

GB-37

GB-38

GB-39

GB-40

GB-41

GB-44

GB-37 Bright Light
光明 *Guang Ming*

Luo-passage point.

Effect Activates the channel, eliminates wind-damp, supports the eyes, draws fire downward.

Indications Pain, neuralgia, paresthesia in the lower leg and knee, pain in the chest area, eye disorders. Brings light in situations of self-abandonment.

Localization On the anterior edge of the fibula on a line between the lateral malleolus and the head of the fibula, at the height of the beginning of the distal third of the lower leg, where the cranial branch of the lateral saphenous vein runs across the lower leg.

Technique To a depth of about 0.3 cun; oblique insertion downward.

GB-38 *Yang* Assistance
阳辅 *Yang Fu*

Fire point, sedation point.

Effect Subdues liver *yang*, clears heat, eliminates damp-heat.

Indications Pain in the hind legs and joints, possibly with swelling; axillary lymphadenitis. Restores the fire quality of playfulness and spontaneity.

Localization 4 cun above the tip of the lateral malleolus, on the anterior edge of the fibula.

Technique To a depth of about 0.3 cun; perpendicular insertion.

GB-39 Suspended Bell
悬钟 *Xuan Zhong*

Hui-meeting point for the marrow.

Effect Promotes essence, nourishes the marrow and the bones, eliminates wind-damp, clears heat in the gallbladder, activates the channel.

Indications Problems of the marrow (brain and spinal cord), epilepsy, disturbed blood production, paralysis in the hind legs, swelling and inflammation in the ankle joint, stiffness and pain in the neck, *bi* (impediment) syndrome with wind-damp, kidney *yin* deficiency. For a weakened internal rhythm.

Localization 3 cun above the tip of the lateral malleolus, in a depression between the posterior edge of the fibula and the tendons of the long and short peroneal muscles, across from SP-6.

Technique To a depth of about 0.2 cun; perpendicular insertion.

GB

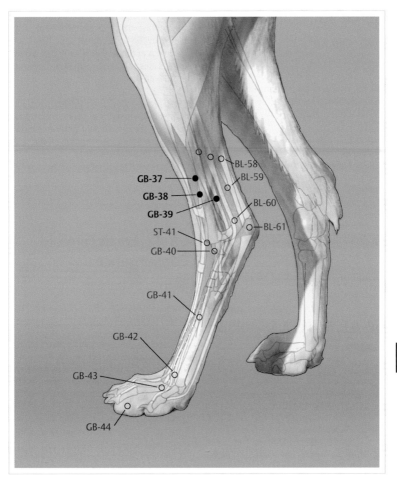

GB-40 Hill Ruins

丘墟 *Qiu Xu*

Yuan-source point.

Effect Supports the smooth flow of liver *qi*, clears damp-heat from the gallbladder, activates the channel.

Indications Pain and swelling in the ankle joint; biliary colic, possibly with stones; hepatopathy; muscle spasms; axillary lymphadenitis. Strengthens the psychological aspect of the gallbladder in cases of internal confusion and disorientation.

Localization Dorsolateral on the ankle joint, distal to the lateral malleolus.

Technique To a depth of about 0.2 cun; perpendicular insertion.

GB-41 Foot Overlooking Tears

足临泣 *Zu Lin Qi*

Shu-stream point, wood point, opener of the girdling vessel (*dai mai*).

Effect Supports the smooth flow of liver *qi*, transforms phlegm and resolves knots, supports the lateral rib area and thorax, connects the lower burner.

Indications Vaginitis; cystitis; urethritis; conjunctivitis; mastitis; swollen lymph nodes; localized problems in the dorsal metatarsus; damp *bi* (impediment) syndrome in the head, throat, hip, and knee; weakness of the hind leg; lumbago; ischialgia. Relaxes the diaphragm and draws out bottled-up rage.

Localization Dorsal on the hind leg, in a depression distal to the connection between the fourth and fifth metatarsal bones, lateral to the tendon of the long extensor muscle of the toes.

Technique To a depth of about 1 cun; oblique insertion in a plantar and distal direction.

GB-42 Earth Fivefold Convergence

地五会 *Di Wu Hui*

Effect Distributes liver *qi*, clears heat from the gallbladder.

Indications Swelling and pain in the armpit area and dorsal hind leg, damp *bi* in the hind toes, mastitis. Stabilizes and coordinates movements, also in the figurative sense.

Localization Dorsal on the hind leg, between the heads of the fourth and fifth metatarsal bones.

Technique To a depth of about 0.2 cun; oblique insertion in a distal direction.

GB

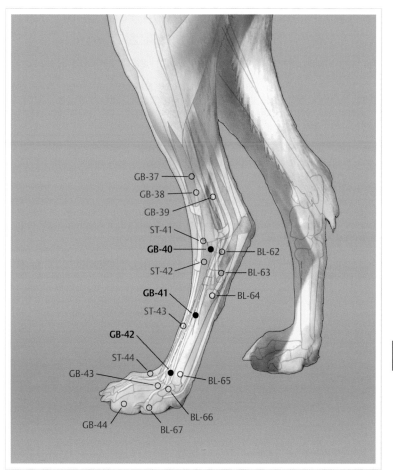

GB-43 Pinched Ravine

侠溪 *Xia Xi*

Ying-brook point, water point, supplementing point.

Effect Subdues liver *yan*; supports the head, eyes, and ears; clears damp-heat and resolves swellings.

Indications Fever, pain in the chest region, conjunctivitis, otitis, mastitis in the thoracic region. Creates prudent courage, also in difficult situations.

Localization Proximal to the digital fold, between the fourth and fifth metatarsophalangeal joints.

Technique To a depth of about 0.2 cun; perpendicular insertion.

GB-44 Foot Orifice *Yin*

足窍阴 *Zu Qiao Yin*

Jing-well point, metal point.

Effect Subdues liver *yang*; clears heat; supports the eyes, head, and lateral rib region; calms the spirit in states of agitation.

Indications Fever; eye disorders; sudden deafness; in conjunction with GB-11, it opens up any sense of pathogenic fullness in deficiency cases; gallbladder inflammation; states of shock; difficulty breathing; laryngopharyngitis; mastitis of the thoracic glands, when overstrain leads to stereotypical actions.

Localization Proximolateral to the claw fold of the fourth toe of the hind leg.

Technique To a depth of about 0.1 cun; oblique insertion in a proximal direction.

GB

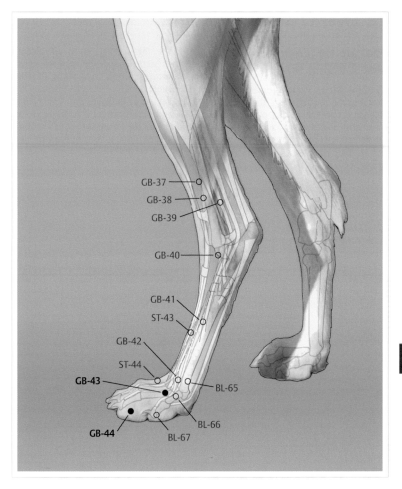

GB-37
GB-38
GB-39
GB-40
GB-41
ST-43
GB-42
ST-44
GB-43
BL-65
GB-44
BL-66
BL-67

22 Liver Channel

Foot *Jue Yin* (*Zu Jue Yin Gan Mai* 足厥阴肝脉)

The liver channel starts its external course lateral to the second toe of the hind paw, ascends across the medial malleolus and the medial side of the leg, and runs around the genital area to the lateral abdomen, to end at point LR-14 in the sixth intercostal space.

From the lumbar area, an internal branch runs around the stomach before connecting with the liver and gallbladder. From here, it continues on through the diaphragm, sends branches into the abdominal and rib areas, and ascends to the throat, into the nasopharynx, and into the eyes. From there, it runs upward to meet the governing vessel (*du mai*) at point GV-20.

LR

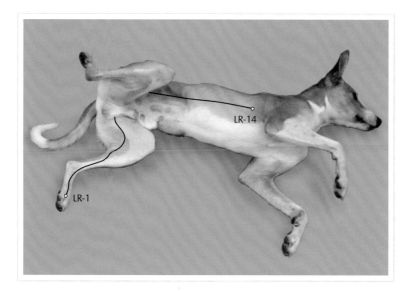

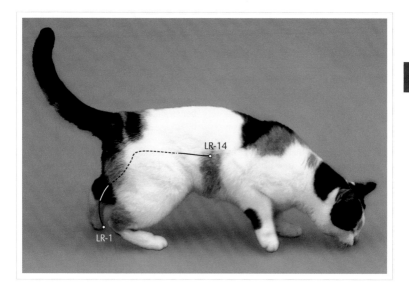

LR

LR-1 Large Pile
大敦 *Da Dun*

Jing-well point, wood point.

Effect   Resolves damp-heat, promotes the smooth flow of liver *qi*, restores consciousness, stops uterine bleeding, supports the genitals, helps with urination.

Indications   Pain in the genitals and inguinal region, swelling in the scrotum, abdominal pain, urinary incontinence. Strengthens self-confidence.

Localization   On the lateral edge of the second toe of the hind paw, dorsolateral nail fold.

Technique   To a depth of about 0.2 cun; perpendicular insertion.

LR-2 Moving Between
行间 *Xing Jian*

Ying brook point, fire point, sedation point.

Effect   Clears liver fire, calms liver *yang* and liver wind, cools blood, stanches bleeding.

Indications   Eye diseases, spasms, constipation, headache, insomnia, cough with pain below the ribs, hepatopathies, irritability, aggressiveness; to balance out the emotions.

Localization   On the hind paw medially on the second toe, distal to the metatarsophalangeal joint, in the middle between the dorsal and medial aspects of the bone.

Technique   To a depth of about 0.3 cun; oblique insertion in a caudodistal direction.

LR-3 Supreme Surge
太冲 *Tai Chong*

Shu-stream point, *yuan*-source point, earth point.

Effect   Calms liver *yang*, calms liver (*gan*) excess, dispels internal wind, promotes the smooth flow of liver *qi*, calms the spirit, calms spasms, nourishes liver blood, clears the head and eyes, regulates the lower burner.

Indications   Liver and gallbladder problems, muscle spasms, muscle pain due to deposits of toxic substances, headache, epilepsy, eye problems, tendency to anxiety and insecurity, impatience, vertigo, coxarthrosis and hip joint dysplasia, urogenital disorders.

Localization   On the hind paw between the second and third toes, slightly underneath half the length of the metatarsal bones on the widest place between the bones.

Technique   To a depth of about 0.8 cun; oblique insertion in a caudodistal direction.

 Contraindicated during pregnancy.

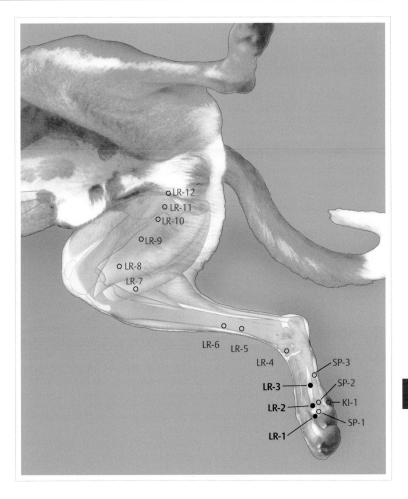

LR

LR-4 Mound Center

中封 *Zhong Feng*

Jing-river point, metal point.

Effect Promotes the smooth flow of liver *qi* in the lower burner, clears congested heat in the liver channel.

Indications Ankle joint problems, contractions in the tendons, pain in the external genitals, hernias. Channels decision-making processes.

Localization On the ankle joint, 1 cun anterior to the medial malleolus, in a depression between the long extensor muscles of the toes and the tibialis cranialis muscles.

Technique To a depth of about 0.3 cun; perpendicular insertion.

LR-5 Woodworm Canal

蠡沟 *Li Gou*

Luo-network point.

Effect Promotes the smooth flow of liver *qi*, eliminates damp-heat from the lower burner, supports the genitals, removes plum-pit *qi* (the *luo* channel begins at this point and encircles the genitals).

Indications Special effect on the genital area in all cases of liver *qi* stagnation, with signs such as a sensation like a plum pit in the throat, abdominal distention, pain during urination, urinary retention, lumbar pain, itching, hepatopathies with occasional light-colored stools, and itching with restrained aggression.

Localization On the medial edge of the tibia, 2 cun above the medial malleolus.

Technique To a depth of about 0.3 cun; perpendicular insertion.

LR-6 Central Metropolis

中都 *Zhong Du*

Xi-cleft point.

Effect Promotes the smooth flow of liver *qi*, regulates the lower burner, removes dampness, regulates blood.

Indications Urogenital problems, pain in the lower abdomen, uterine bleeding, unstoppable diarrhea. Helpful for staying centered in conditions marked by pain.

Localization On the medial edge of the tibia, 3 cun above the medial malleolus.

Technique To a depth of about 0.3 cun; perpendicular insertion.

LR

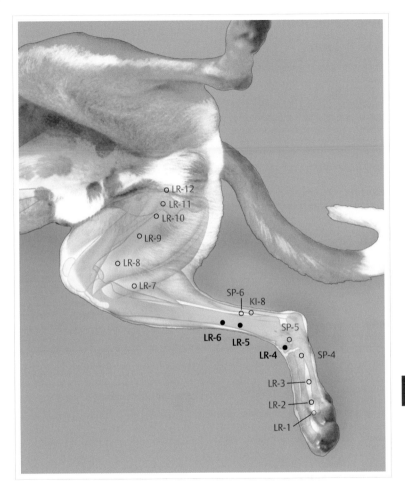

LR

LR-7 Knee Joint

膝关 *Xi Guan*

Effect Disperses wind-damp, supports the knees.

Indications Pain on the inside of the knee joint, urogenital problems, pain in the lower abdomen. For extreme stubbornness.

Localization Caudodistal to the medial condyle of the tibia, 1 cun caudal to SP-9.

Technique To a depth of about 0.5 cun; perpendicular insertion.

LR-8 Spring at the Bend

曲泉 *Qu Quan*

He-sea point, water point, supplementing point.

Effect Promotes the bladder, eliminates damp-heat from the lower burner, nourishes blood and *yin*, relaxes the tendons, supports the genitals and uterus.

Indications Pain in the urogenital tract, weakened libido, pain in the medial knee region and in the groin, changing consistency of stools, bright-colored stools with itching, hepatopathy, impaired vision,

fatigue. Promotes constancy and flexibility, calms down exaggerated heated reactions.

Localization Behind the medial condyle of the femur, proximal to the medial knee fold in front of the attachment of the semimembranous and semitendinous muscles.

Technique To a depth of about 1 cun; perpendicular insertion.

LR-9 *Yin* Bladder

阴包 *Yin Bao*

Effect Regulates the lower burner.

Indications Pain on the inside of the thigh, dysuria, irregular estrous cycles.

Localization Central on the inner thigh between the bellies of the gracilis and sartorius muscles, proximal to the medial epicondyle of the femur at the level where the femoral artery becomes palpable.

Technique To a depth of about 1 cun; perpendicular insertion.

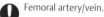 Femoral artery/vein.

LR

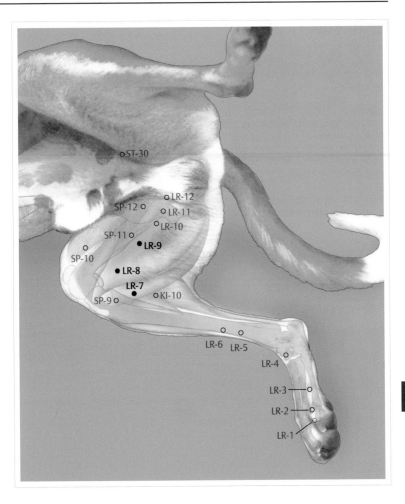

LR-10 Foot Five *Li*
足五里 *Zu Wu Li*

Effect   Clears damp-heat, especially in the lower burner.

Indications   Pain on the inside of the thigh, hip pain, lumbago, dysuria, itching in the genital area.

Localization   Central on the inside of the thigh, about 2 cun distal to ST-30.

Technique   To a depth of about 1 cun; perpendicular insertion.

 Femoral artery/vein.

LR-11 Yin Corner
阴廉 *Yin Lian*

Effect   Supports the uterus.

Indications   Irregular estrous cycles; sterility in bitches; pain in the inner thigh, in the lower abdomen, and in the hip joints. Relaxes the lower body and the attitude toward sexuality.

Localization   Central on the inside of the thigh, about 1 cun distal to ST-30.

Technique   To a depth of about 0.5 cun; perpendicular insertion.

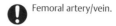 Femoral artery/vein.

LR-12 Urgent Pulse
急脉 *Ji Mai*

Effect   Supports the lower burner, removes cold from the liver channel.

Indications   Pain in the lower abdomen, in the inguinal area, and on the external genitals. Helps when internal pressure is discharged as hypersexuality.

Localization   Central on the inside of the thigh, roughly in the area of the inguinal canal.

Technique   To a depth of about 0.3 cun; perpendicular insertion (preferably treated only with moxa).

 Femoral artery/vein.

LR

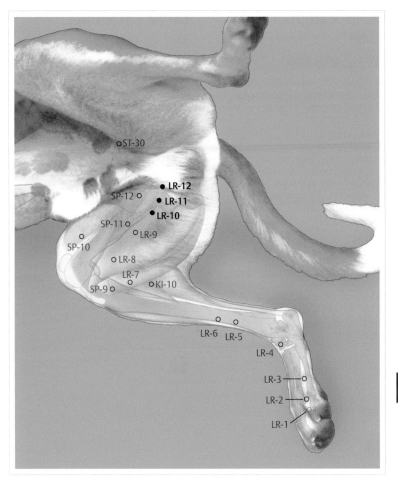

LR-13 Camphorwood Gate

章门 *Zhang Men*

Mu alarm point of the spleen, *hui*-meeting point of the viscera, intersection point with the gallbladder channel.

Effect Supports the harmonious flow of *qi*, supports the transformation functions of the spleen, disperses and transforms dampness, resolves food stagnation, regulates the center and lower burners, moves *qi* upward to the lung and downward to the kidneys, harmonizes the liver and spleen.

Indications Abdominal pain, diarrhea, vomiting, hepatopathies, cholecystopathies, cholangiopathies, gastroduodenitis, pancreatitis, fatigue during convalescence, intercostal neuralgia. Helps to release an old grudge and have a new beginning.

Localization On the lateral wall of the abdomen, at the transition to the cartilage portion of the second to last, that is, 12th, rib.

Technique To a depth of about 0.3 cun; tangential insertion.

 Risk of pneumothorax.

LR-14 Cycle Gate

期门 *Qi Men*

Mu alarm point of the liver, intersection point with the spleen channel and the *yin* linking vessel (*yin wei mai*).

Effect Supports the smooth flow of liver *qi*, disperses food stagnation, resolves masses, cools blood, harmonizes the liver and stomach.

Indications Muscle problems, painful tense abdomen, intercostal neuralgia, hepatitis, hypogalactia, mastitis, travel sickness, depression due to liver *qi* stagnation.

Localization In the sixth intercostal space or in the seventh from behind, at the height of the costochondral transition of the sixth rib. Alternative descriptions place the point in the 10th intercostal space.

Technique To a depth of about 0.3 cun; tangential insertion.

 Risk of pneumothorax.

LR

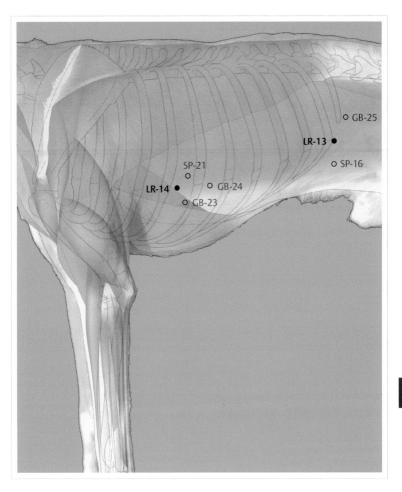

23 Governing Vessel

Governing Vessel
(*Du Mai* 督脉)

The governing vessel starts its external course between the base of the tail and the anus. From there, it runs ventrally under the midline of the tail to its tip, and switches there over to its dorsal midline. It proceeds along the midline of the back to the front to GV-16, from where it enters the brain in the area of the back of the neck. Externally, it continues to ascend across the back of the neck and occiput to the highest point of the skull at GV-20, from where it runs across the forehead and nose to the philtrum, ending at GV-28 inside below the upper lip.

A branch originates in the lower abdomen, runs to the genitals, circumvents the anus, and proceeds inside the spinal column to the kidneys. Another branch ascends through the navel to the heart, from there on through the neck around the muzzle, and then upward to below the eyes. A third branch, after reaching the surface at BL-1, follows a path bilateral to the bladder channel across the forehead and enters the brain.

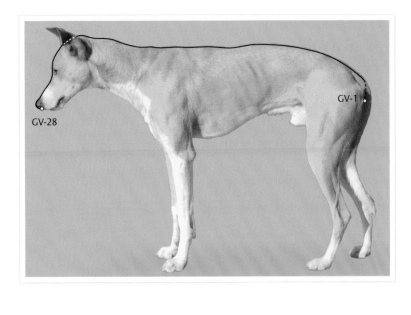

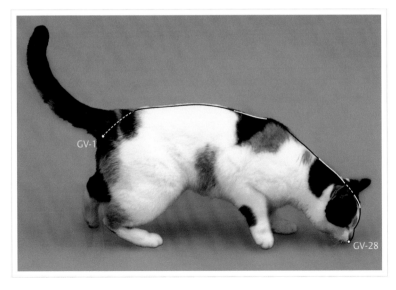

GV-1 Long Strong

长强 *Chang Qiang*

Intersection point with the controlling vessel (*ren mai*) and the kidney and gallbladder channels, *luo*-passage point of the governing vessel (*du mai*).

Effect Regulates the intestines, activates the channel, resolves damp-heat, calms the spirit.

Indications Swellings, rectal prolapse, weak sphincter muscle, anal sac inflammation, anal eczema, meconium retention, gastrointestinal problems, urogenital problems, dysfunctions of the hind legs, all problems of the governing vessel or spinal column, pain in the caudal back, constipation, diarrhea, tenesmus.

Localization In a depression between the anus and the ventral base of the tail, between the coccygeal muscle and the sphincter muscles of the anus.

Technique To a depth of about 2 cun; perpendicular insertion.

GV

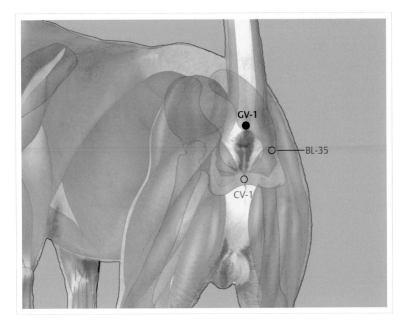

GV-2 Lumbar Transport

腰俞 *Yao Shu*

Effect Disperses internal wind, calms spasms and twitching, strengthens the posterior back.

Indications Weakness of the hind leg, lumbago, diarrhea, rectal prolapse, urinary incontinence, urogenital problems.

Localization Dorsal in the sacrococcygeal space.

Technique To a depth of about 1.5 cun; perpendicular insertion.

GV

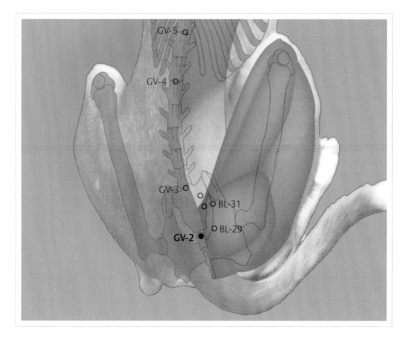

GV-3 Lower Hundred Convergences

下百会 *Xiao Bai Hui*

GV-3 is variously located and named in different sources. The localization of GV-3 varies in the intercostal spaces of the fourth to seventh lumbar vertebrae and in the lumbosacral space. Sometimes, it is also referred to as GV-3–1 to GV-3–4 because evidently the acupuncture point effect has been found everywhere here.

In this acupuncture point atlas, the description of GV-3 places it in the lumbosacral space. The points between the spinous processes of the lumbar spinal column have a comparable but weaker effect.

Effect Supplements kidney *yang*, strengthens the lower back and hind legs, regulates the lower burner, expels wind-damp.

Indications Pain in the lower back, especially when radiating into the hind legs; spondyloses in the lumbar spine; weakness and atrophy in the hind legs, for example, cauda equina syndrome; sprain in the hind leg; lumbago; hip joint arthritis; discopathy; impotence; retained placenta; endometritis; arthritis in the hip joint; colic; dilated stomach.

Localization In the lumbosacral space.

Technique To a depth of about 1.5 cun; perpendicular insertion.

GV-4 Life Gate

命门 *Ming Men*

Effect Supplements *yang*, especially kidney *yang*, supplements original (*yuan*) *qi*, supplements the kidney's fluid metabolism, nourishes the essence, strengthens the lumbar area and the knees, removes internal cold in cases of *yang* deficiency, clears heat, regulates the governing vessel (*du mai*).

Indications All kidney problems, pain in the lower back and knees, discopathy, spondylosis, disorders in the urogenital system, infertility, conditions of sexual deficiency, exhaustion, intestinal problems with cold and/or *yang* deficiency, sprain and rheumatism in the hind leg, problems in the urogenital system and intestinal area.

Localization Dorsal between the second and third lumbar vertebrae.

Technique To a depth of about 1.5 cun; perpendicular insertion.

GV

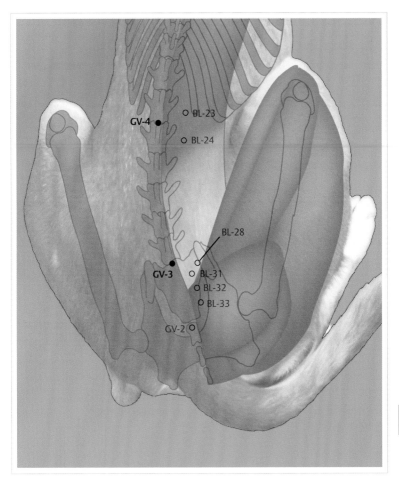

GV-5 Suspended Pivot
悬枢 *Xuan Shu*

Effect   Supports the lumbar spine and the lower burner.

Indications   Enteritis; diarrhea; pain in the lumbar spine, hip, and thighs; bleeding.

Localization   Medially between the last thoracic and the first lumbar vertebrae.

Technique   To a depth of about 1.5 cun; perpendicular insertion.

GV-6 Spinal Center
脊中 *Ji Zhong*

Effect   Eliminates dampness, strengthens the spleen.

Indications   Bleeding after surgery, epistaxis, hematuria, diarrhea, pain in the lumbar area.

Localization   Medially between the 12th and 13th thoracic vertebrae.

Technique   To a depth of about 1.5 cun; perpendicular insertion.

GV-7 Central Pivot
中枢 *Zhong Shu*

Effect   Supports the center burner and the spinal column.

Indications   Stomach pain, localized pain, bleeding after surgery, epistaxis, hematuria.

Localization   Medially between the 11th and 12th thoracic vertebrae.

Technique   To a depth of about 1.5 cun; perpendicular insertion.

GV-8 Sinew Contraction
筋缩 *Jin Suo*

Effect   Soothes the liver, calms the spirit and wind.

Indications   Epilepsy, muscle cramps, spasms, stiffness in the neck, stomach cramps.

Localization   Medially between the ninth and 10th thoracic vertebrae.

Technique   To a depth of about 1.5 cun; perpendicular insertion.

GV

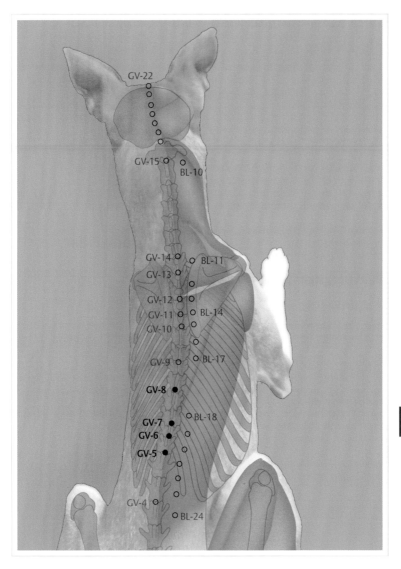

GV-9 Consummate *Yang*

至阳 *Zhi Yang*

Effect Regulates the liver and gallbladder, opens up the thorax and diaphragm, moves the *qi*, eliminates damp-heat, strengthens the spleen.

Indications Hypochondriac pain, intercostal neuralgia, icterus, lack of energy.

Localization Medially between the seventh and eighth thoracic vertebrae. Alternatively, it is also described as being located behind the 10th thoracic vertebra.

Technique To a depth of about 1.5 cun; perpendicular insertion.

GV-10 Spirit Tower

灵台 *Ling Tai*

Effect Clears heat and detoxifies, relieves coughing and panting.

Indications Localized back pain, bronchitis, asthma, pneumonia.

Localization Between the fifth and sixth thoracic vertebrae. Alternatively, it is also described as being located behind the seventh thoracic vertebra.

Technique To a depth of about 1.5 cun; perpendicular insertion.

GV-11 Spirit Path

神道 *Shen Dao*

Effect Calms the spirit, regulates the heart and lung, clears heat, calms wind.

Indications Asthma, cough, heart problems, anxiety with shortness of breath, back pain, spondyloses.

Localization Medially between the fourth and fifth thoracic vertebrae.

Technique To a depth of about 1.5 cun; perpendicular insertion.

GV-12 Body Pillar

身柱 *Shen Zhu*

Effect Supplements lung *qi*, clears heat from the heart and lungs, removes wind, calms the spirit.

Indications Stiffness and pain in the lumbar region and back, cough, bronchitis.

Localization Medially between the third and fourth thoracic vertebrae.

Technique To a depth of about 1.5 cun; perpendicular insertion.

GV

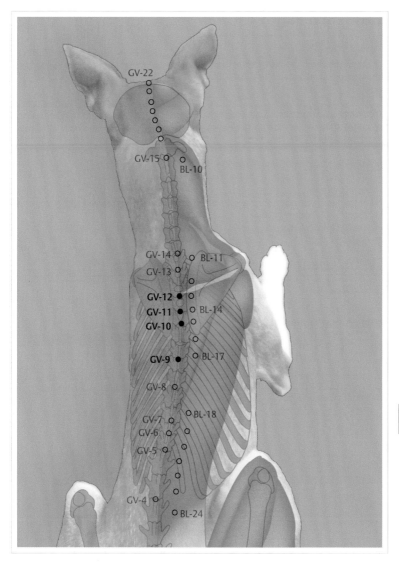

GV-13 Kiln Path

陶道 *Tao Dao*

Effect Clears heat, relaxes the exterior, regulates the bladder and the governing vessel.

Indications Cough, asthma, enterospasm, torticollis, stiffness in the spinal column, febrile disorders.

Localization In a depression between the spinous processes of the first and second thoracic vertebrae.

Technique To a depth of about 1.5 cun; perpendicular insertion.

GV-14 Great Hammer

大椎 *Da Zhui*

Intersection point with the six *yang* channels, a point on the sea of *qi*.

Effect Dispels wind-heat, clears the brain, calms the spirit, supplements *yang*, regulates food (*gu*) and defense (*wei*) *qi*, clears heat, supplements deficient states, strengthens the surface.

Indications Neck problems, disorders of the cervical spine, occipital neuralgias, infectious diseases with rhythmic occurrence, respiratory tract problems, asthma, cough, cold, fever, heat stroke, chills, brain, eczema, lack of energy, epilepsy.

Localization In a depression on the dorsal midline, between the seventh cervical and the first thoracic vertebrae.

Technique To a depth of about 1.5 cun; perpendicular insertion.

GV-15 Mute's Gate

哑门 *Ya Men*

Effect Intersection point with the *yang* linking vessel (*yang wei mai*), a point on the sea of *qi*.

Indications Stroke, torticollis, occipital neuralgia, convulsions, cervical syndrome.

Localization Medially between atlas and axis.

Technique To a depth of about 1 cun; insertion in a cranioventral direction.

GV

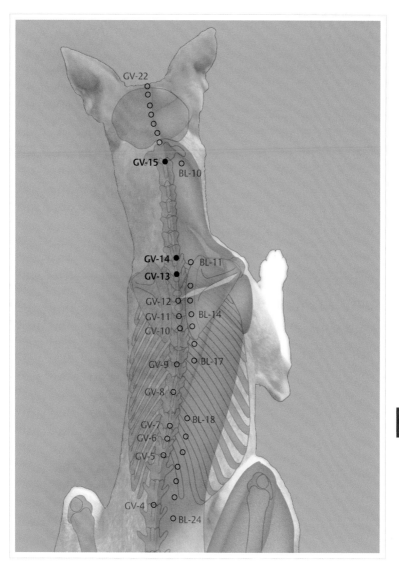

GV-16 Wind House

风府 *Feng Fu*

Intersection point with the *yang* linking vessel (*yang wei mai*), a point on the sea of marrow.

Effect Expels wind, clears the spirit, promotes the brain and back of the neck.

Indications Stiff neck, epistaxis, pharyngitis, cold, encephalitis, hypothalamic problems, tetanus, wind apoplexy. Calms the mind. With GV-20 for epilepsy.

Localization On the dorsal midline, directly below the occipital protuberances.

Technique To a depth of about 0.5 cun; oblique insertion toward posterior.

GV-17 Brain's Door

脑户 *Nao Hu*

Intersection point with the bladder channel.

Effect Eliminates wind, calms the spirit, moves *qi* along the channel.

Indications Epilepsy; pain in the head and neck, possibly with dizziness.

Localization On the dorsal midline, directly below the occipital protuberances.

Technique To a depth of about 1 cun; oblique tangential insertion in a rostral direction.

GV-18 Unyielding Space

强间 *Qiang Jian*

Effect Eliminates wind, calms the spirit, moves *qi* along the channel.

Indications Headache, neck pain, epileptiform seizures.

Localization On the dorsal midline of the head, rostral to the occipital protuberances.

Technique To a depth of about 0.5 cun; oblique insertion in a rostral direction.

GV

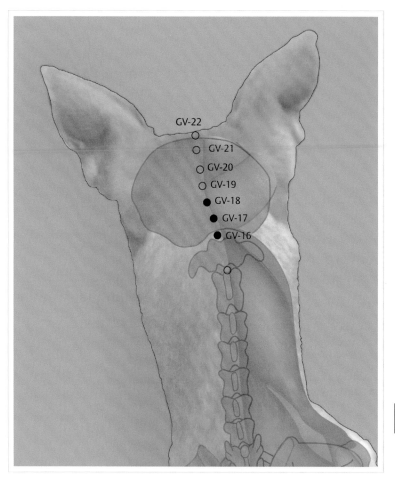

GV-19 Behind the Vertex

后顶 *Hou Ding*

Effect Eliminates wind, calms the spirit, moves *qi* along the channel.

Indications States of excitement, epilepsy, insomnia, strong panting, impaired vision.

Localization Approximately halfway between GV-20 and GV-18.

Technique To a depth of about 0.5 cun; oblique insertion toward the front.

GV-20 Hundred Convergences

百会 *Bai Hui*

Effect Promotes the function of the spleen to transport *qi* upward, strong effect in promoting *yang*, calms wind and the mind, counteracts prolapse, supports the brain, clears and stimulates the spirit, nourishes the sea of marrow.

Indications Rectal and uterine prolapse, incontinence, polydipsia, convulsions, ear and eye problems, stimulating immunity, calming, strokes, epilepsy, circulatory disorders in the brain, tetanus, allergic shock.

Localization On the dorsal midline of the head where it intersects with a line between the rostral edges of the bases of the ears, slightly caudal to the highest point on the head.

Technique To a depth of about 0.5 cun; slightly oblique insertion in a rostral direction.

GV-21 Before the Vertex

前顶 *Qian Ding*

Effect Eliminates wind, supports the head.

Indications Severe rhinitis, epilepsy.

Localization Central on the skull cap, vertically above the bases of the ears about 0.5 cun in front of LG-20.

Technique To a depth of about 0.5 cun; slightly oblique insertion in a rostral direction.

GV-22 Fontanel Meeting

囟会 *Xin Hui*

Effect Eliminates wind, supports the nose.

Indications Lost sense of smell, nasal discharge, headache.

Localization About 0.3 cun cranial to GV-21.

Technique To a depth of about 0.5 cun; oblique insertion in a rostral direction.

GV

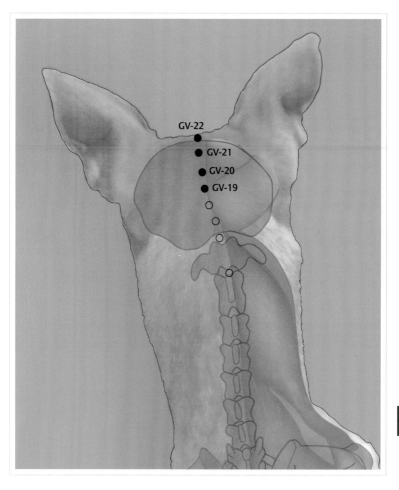

GV-23 Upper Star

上星 *Shang Xing*

Effect Eliminates wind and dampness, calms the spirit, supports the nose and eyes.

Indications Sinusitis, rhinitis, eye problems, swollen scalp.

Localization Centrally on the skull cap between GV-22 and GV-24.

Technique To a depth of about 0.5 cun; oblique insertion in a rostral direction.

GV-24 Spirit Court

神庭 *Shen Ting*

Intersection point with the bladder channel.

Effect Calms the spirit; supports the brain, head, eyes, and nose; eliminates wind.

Indications Fear, convulsions, tetanus, encephalitis, sinusitis, rhinitis, eye problems.

Localization On the dorsal midline of the skull cap 1 cun dorsal to the inner corner of the eye.

Technique To a depth of about 0.5 cun; oblique insertion in a rostral direction.

GV-25 White Bone-Hole

素髎 *Su Liao*

Effect Supports the nose.

Indications Rhinitis, lung congestion, cerebral hyperemia, unconsciousness, asphyxia in newborns.

Localization On the nose, dorsal to GV-26, at the point where it meets the tendon of the levator labii maxillaris, on the transition from hairy to hairless skin.

Technique To a depth of about 0.2 cun; perpendicular insertion.

GV

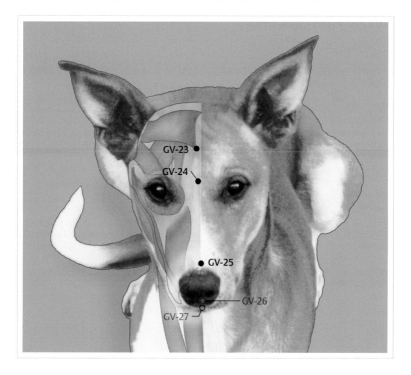

GV-26 Human Center

人中 *Ren Zhong*

Intersection point with the large intestine and stomach channels.

Effect Restores consciousness, calms the spirit, increases brain activity, increases heart rate and respiratory frequency, significantly increases endorphin release, clears the senses, eliminates wind, supports the lumbar spine.

Indications Emergency point, point for resuscitation, shock, epilepsy, postanesthetic apnea, neonatal asphyxia, coma, facial nerve paresis, cramping of the jaw muscles.

Localization In the philtrum at the end of the reversed "T."

Technique To a depth of about 0.3 cun; perpendicular insertion.

GV-27 Extremity of the Mouth

兑端 *Dui Duan*

Effect Supports the mouth and chin, clears heat, produces fluid, calms the spirit.

Indications Toothache, inflammations of the oral mucosa.

Localization Centrally on the upper lip, on the transition from the hairy skin to the mucosa.

Technique To a depth of about 0.3 cun; perpendicular insertion.

GV

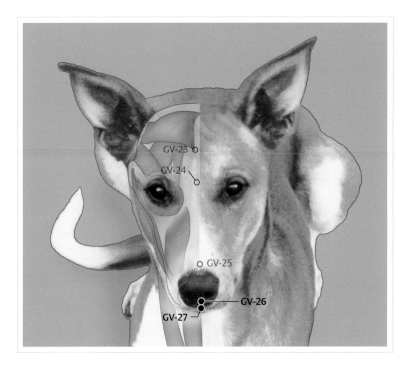

GV-28 Gum Intersection

龈交 *Yin Jiao*

Intersection point with the controlling vessel (*ren mai*) and the stomach (*wei*) channel.

Effect Supports the mouth and chin, clears heat, moves fluids.

Indications Stomatitis, gingivitis, tooth abscesses, digestive disorders, pharyngolaryngitis, constant tearing, nasal discharge.

Localization Inside between the mucosa on the upper lip and the edge of the upper gums.

Technique To a depth of about 0.3 cun; perpendicular insertion.

GV

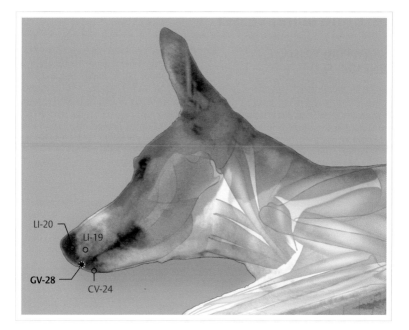

24 Controlling Vessel

Controlling Vessel
(*Ren Mai* 任脉)

The controlling vessel originates in the uterus in female and in the lower abdomen in male animals. From there, it emerges to the surface at CV-1 between the anus and the vulva or scrotum. The controlling vessel continues along the midline across the lower and upper abdomen, sternum, throat, and jaw from the back to the front, to the base of the tongue. It ends at CV-24 on the lower lip. An internal branch runs around the mouth, connects to the governing vessel at GV-2, and ends at ST-1 below the eye.

An additional branch originates in the lesser pelvis, enters the spinal column, and ascends along the back.

CV

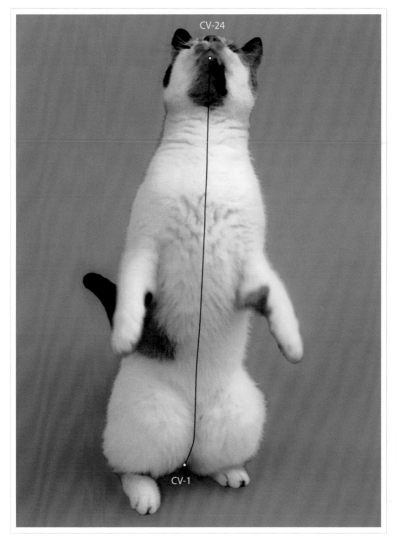

CV-1 Meeting of *Yin*

会阴 *Hui Yin*

Intersection point with the thoroughfare vessel (*chong mai*) and governing vessel (*du mai*).

Effect Nourishes and regulates *yin* and essence; removes damp-heat, especially from the urogenital area; calms the spirit.

Indications Urethritis, pain in the uterus, uterine prolapse, rectal prolapse, urinary retention, menstrual disorders, vaginitis, anal sac inflammation, weakness in the lumbosacral area and hindquarters.

Localization Centrally on the midline, between anus and vulva in female animals and between anus and scrotum in male animals.

Technique To a depth of about 1 cun; perpendicular insertion.

> The points CV-2 to CV-8 are located on the ventral midline between the pelvic symphysis and the navel. This area is divided into five sections, and each section is defined as 1 cun. The following information on localization refers to this definition.

CV-2 Curved Bone

曲骨 *Qu Gu*

Intersection point with the liver channel.

Effect Regulates the lower burner, supports urination and the kidneys, warms the kidneys.

Indications Irregular estrous cycle, impotence, endometritis, hernias, urinary retention.

Localization In the middle of the cranial border of the symphysis.

Technique To a depth of about 1 cun; perpendicular insertion.

CV-3 Central Pole

中极 *Zhong Ji*

Mu-alarm point of the bladder; intersection point with the spleen, liver, and kidney channels.

Effect Regulates the uterus, draws out damp-heat, supports the bladder and regulates *qi* transformation, resolves stagnations, supports the lower burner, strengthens the kidneys.

Indications Problems in the urogenital system; problems with urination and delivery; infertility, especially in bitches; retained placenta.

Localization On the ventral midline, 4 cun caudal to the navel, 1 cun cranial to the pelvic symphysis.

Technique To a depth of about 0.5 cun; tangential insertion.

 Potential risk of puncturing the abdominal cavity.

CV

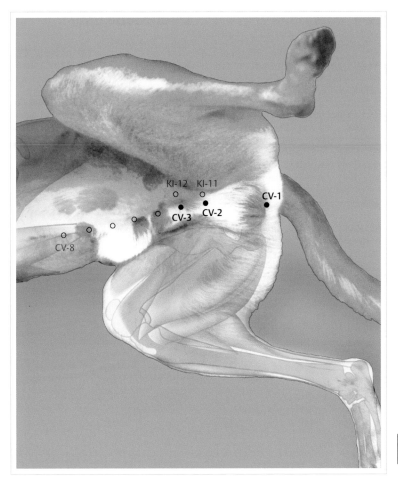

CV

CV-4 Pass Head
关元 *Guan Yuan*

Mu-alarm point of the small intestine; intersection point with the spleen, liver, and kidney channels.

Effect Nourishes blood and *yin*, strengthens *yang*, roots the ethereal (*hun*) soul, supports original (*yuan*) *qi* and essence, supplements and nourishes the kidneys, warms and strengthens the spleen, supports the uterus, regulates the lower burner, regulates the *qi* of the small intestine.

Indications Pain and inflammations in the lower abdomen, tendency to intestinal parasites, bladder infection, diarrhea, irregular estrous cycles, uterine prolapse, hernias, impotence due to exhaustion, general weakness.

Localization On the ventral midline, 3 cun caudal to the navel, 2 cun cranial to the pelvic symphysis.

Technique To a depth of about 0.5 cun; tangential insertion.

 Do not needle during pregnancy! Potential risk of puncturing the abdominal cavity.

CV-5 Stone Gate
石门 *Shi Men*

Mu-alarm point of the triple burner channel.

Effect Strengthens original (*yuan*) *qi*, opens up the waterways by supporting the transformation and excretion of fluids in the lower burner.

Indications Problems of the urogenital system, gastrointestinal problems, ascites, abdominal pain, diarrhea, infertility, lack of appetite, irregular estrous cycle, bladder infection, tendency to edema.

Localization On the ventral midline, 2 cun caudal to the navel, 3 cun cranial to the pelvic symphysis.

Technique To a depth of about 0.5 cun; tangential insertion.

 Potential risk of puncturing the abdominal cavity.

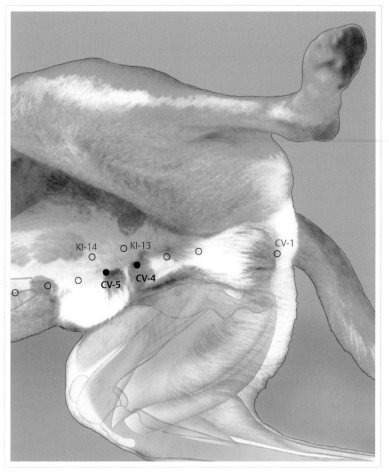

CV-6 Sea of *Qi*

气海 *Qi Hai*

Effect Supplements the kidneys and regulates *qi*, *yang*, and original *qi*; resolves dampness, harmonizes blood.

Indications Weakness of the urethral sphincter, problems in the gastrointestinal tract, in combination with moxa for soft stools, physical and mental exhaustion, weakness of the viscera with *qi* exhaustion, abdominal masses, feeling of pressure in the abdomen, pain and cold sensation below the navel, retracted testicles, to strengthen willpower.

Localization On the ventral midline, 1.5 cun caudal to the navel, 3.5 cun cranial to the pelvic symphysis.

Technique To a depth of about 0.5 cun; tangential insertion.

 Potential risk of puncturing the abdominal cavity.

CV-7 *Yin* Intersection

阴交 *Yin Jiao*

Intersection point with the thoroughfare vessel (*chong mai*) and the kidney channel.

Effect Warms the kidneys, regulates the controlling vessel (*ren mai*) and thoroughfare vessel (*chong mai*), regulates the uterus.

Indications Pain in the abdomen, hernias, pain in the navel, dysuria, uterine pathologies, nymphomania, satyriasis, pruritus vulvae.

Localization On the ventral midline, 1 cun caudal to the navel, 4 cun cranial to the pelvic symphysis.

Technique To a depth of about 0.5 cun; tangential insertion.

 Potential risk of puncturing the abdominal cavity.

CV-8 Spirit Gate Tower

神阙 *Shen Que*

Effect Strengthens spleen *yang*; supplements, warms, and stabilizes *yang*; remediates collapse.

Indications *Yang qi* collapse; problems of the gastrointestinal tract; abdominal pain, specifically chronic diarrhea; sterility in bitches; extreme weakness; wind collapse.

Localization In the center of the navel.

Technique Needling is contraindicated. Moxa or massage is preferable.

 Potential risk of puncturing the abdominal cavity.

CV

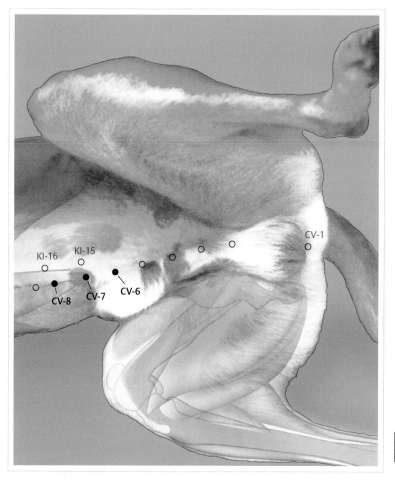

CV

The points CV-9 to CV-15 are located on the ventral midline between the navel and the xiphoid process. This area is divided into seven sections, each section being defined as 1 cun. The following information refers to this definition.

CV-9 Water Divide

水分 *Shui Fen*

Effect Promotes fluid transformation, opens the waterways, eliminates dampness and accumulations.

Indications Dysuria, severe abdominal pain with distention, purulent processes everywhere, edemas, ascites.

Localization On the ventral midline, 1 cun cranial to the navel.

Technique To a depth of about 0.5 cun; tangential insertion.

 Potential risk of puncturing the abdominal cavity.

CV-10 Lower Stomach Duct

下脘 *Xia Wan*

Intersection point with the spleen channel.

Effect Regulates stomach *qi*, supplements the spleen, relieves feed stagnation.

Indications Feeling of fullness in the abdomen, no desire to eat, dysentery.

Localization On the ventral midline, 2 cun cranial to the navel.

Technique To a depth of about 0.5 cun; tangential insertion.

 Potential risk of puncturing the abdominal cavity.

CV-11 Interior Strengthening

建里 *Jian Li*

Effect Harmonizes the center and regulates *qi*.

Indications Abdominal pain, mastitis, swellings.

Localization On the ventral midline, 3 cun cranial to the navel.

Technique To a depth of about 0.5 cun; tangential insertion.

Potential risk of puncturing the abdominal cavity.

CV

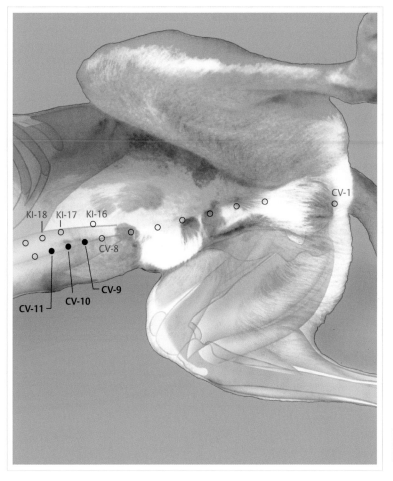

CV-12 Central Stomach Duct

中脘 *Zhong Wan*

Mu-alarm point of the stomach; *hui*-meeting point of the bowels; intersection point with the small intestine, triple burner, and stomach channels.

Effect Influential point for all *yang* conditions, supports the stomach, lowers rebellious *qi*, promotes the splenic functions of transport and transformation, dispels and transforms dampness, disperses food stagnation.

Indications Gastrointestinal problems, weakened digestion, gastroduodenal ulcers, colic, diarrhea, infectious gastrointestinal diseases.

Localization On the ventral midline, halfway between the xiphoid process and the navel.

Technique To a depth of about 0.5 cun; tangential insertion.

 Potential risk of puncturing the abdominal cavity.

CV-13 Upper Stomach Duct

上脘 *Shang Wan*

Intersection point with the stomach and small intestine channels.

Effect Harmonizes the stomach, lowers rebellious *qi*, regulates the heart.

Indications Mastitis in the cranial teats, swelling, vomiting, abdominal pain, weakened digestion, abdominal masses.

Localization On the ventral midline, 5 cun cranial to the navel.

Technique To a depth of about 0.5 cun; tangential insertion.

 Potential risk of puncturing the abdominal cavity.

CV

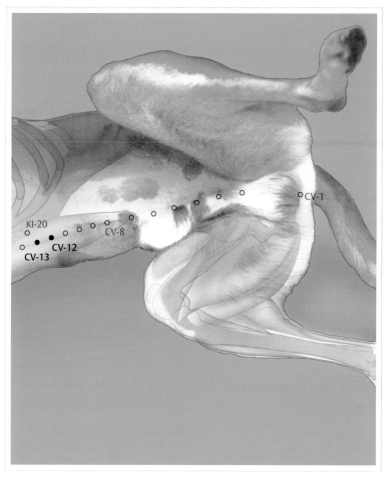

CV-14 Great Tower Gate

巨阙 *Ju Que*

Mu-alarm point of the heart.

Effect Supports the stomach and lowers rebellious *qi*, calms the spirit, regulates the heart, lowers lung *qi* and frees the thorax, transforms phlegm, moves *qi* along the channel.

Indications Stress-related problems of the heart and stomach, cardiac arrhythmia, fear, stomach disorders, stomach pain, vomiting, edemas.

Localization On the ventral midline, midway between the xiphoid process and CV-12, one quarter of the distance between the xiphoid process and the navel.

Technique To a depth of about 0.5 cun; tangential insertion toward caudal.

 Potential risk of puncturing the abdominal cavity.

CV-15 Turtledove Tail

鸠尾 *Jiu Wei*

Luo-passage point.

Effect Calms the spirit, supports the heart and original *qi*, lowers lung *qi*.

Indications Gastritis, "reverse sneezing," hiccup, angina, difficulty in swallowing, states of anxiety, epilepsy, regional abdominal pain.

Localization On the ventral midline directly below the xiphoid process.

Technique To a depth of about 0.5 cun; tangential insertion in a caudal direction.

 Potential risk of puncturing the abdominal cavity.

CV-16 Center Palace

中庭 *Zhong Ting*

Effect Lowers rebellious stomach *qi*, frees the thorax.

Indications Nausea, feeling of fullness in the thorax, vomiting after eating, asthmatic bronchitis.

Localization On the transition from the xiphoid process to the body of the sternum.

Technique To a depth of about 0.5 cun; tangential insertion in a caudal direction.

CV

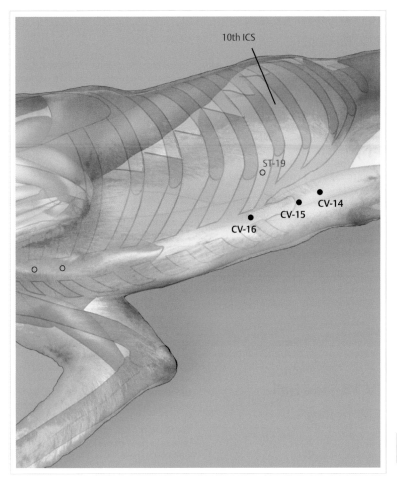

10th ICS

ST-19

CV-14

CV-15

CV-16

CV-17 Chest Center
膻中 *Dan Zhong*

Mu-alarm point of the pericardium; *hui*-meeting point of *qi*, circulation, and the thorax; a point of the sea of *qi*; intersection point with the kidney, spleen, small intestine, and triple burner channels.

Effect Regulates *qi*, supplements center *qi*, stimulates the lung function of the *qi*, lowers rebellion in the lung and stomach, supports the mammary glands and promotes lactation.

Indications Functional problems of the thorax, heart, and lung; phlegm congestion in the lung; epistaxis; mastitis; excessive lactation; swollen teats; anhidrosis.

Localization On the ventral midline above the body of the sternum at the level of the caudal edge of the elbow, by the fourth intercostal space.

Technique To a depth of about 0.5 cun; tangential insertion in a caudal direction.

CV-18 Jade Hall
玉堂 *Yu Tang*

Effect Regulates *qi*, frees the thorax.

Indications Mastitis, swelling, pain in the thorax.

Localization On the ventral midline above the body of the sternum, by the third intercostal space.

Technique To a depth of about 0.3 cun; tangential insertion in a caudal direction.

CV-19 Purple Palace
紫宮 *Zi Gong*

Effect Regulates *qi*, frees the thorax.

Indications Mastitis, swelling, pain in the thorax, cough.

Localization On the ventral midline above the body of the sternum, by the second intercostal space.

Technique To a depth of about 0.3 cun; tangential insertion in a caudal direction.

CV-20 Florid Canopy
华盖 *Hua Gai*

Effect Regulates *qi*, frees the thorax.

Indications Pain in the thorax, cough, asthma, pharyngitis, difficulty swallowing.

Localization On the ventral midline above the body of the sternum, by the first intercostal space.

Technique To a depth of about 0.3 cun; tangential insertion in a caudal direction.

CV

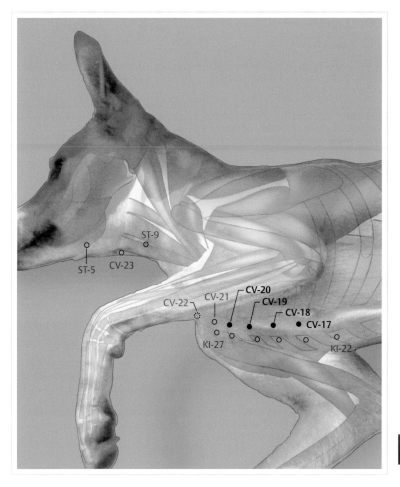

CV-21 Jade Swivel

璇玑 *Xuan Ji*

Effect Regulates *qi*, frees the throat and thorax, lowers lung and stomach *qi*, eliminates food accumulations.

Indications Pain in the chest, cough, asthma, pharyngitis, difficulty in swallowing, nausea, impaired food intake.

Localization On the midline centrally on the manubrium of the sternum.

Technique To a depth of about 0.3 cun; tangential insertion in a caudal direction.

CV-22 Celestial Chimney

天突 *Tian Tu*

Intersection point of the *yin* linking vessel (*yin wei mai*) and the controlling vessel (*ren mai*).

Effect Stimulates the descent of lung *qi*, frees the thorax, eliminates food accumulations, lowers stomach *qi*, cools the throat, clears the voice.

Indications Problems in the upper and lower respiratory tract, esophageal spasms, swelling in the throat area with difficulty in swallowing, local lymphadenitis, swollen thyroid, nervous vomiting, cough, asthma, pharyngitis.

Localization In a depression cranial to the tip of the sternum.

Technique To a depth of about 1 cun; insertion dorsal to the manubrium in a caudal direction.

CV-23 Ridge Spring

廉泉 *Lian Quan*

Intersection point with the *yin* linking vessel (*yin wei mai*).

Effect Promotes the voice, dispels internal wind, clears heat, resolves phlegm, lowers rebellious *qi*.

Indications Pharyngitis, laryngitis, hyoid bone blockage with impaired tongue mobility and difficulty in swallowing, swollen thyroid.

Localization On the ventral midline of the neck, in a depression behind the ventral branch of the hyoid bone.

Technique To a depth of about 0.5 cun; tangential insertion.

CV

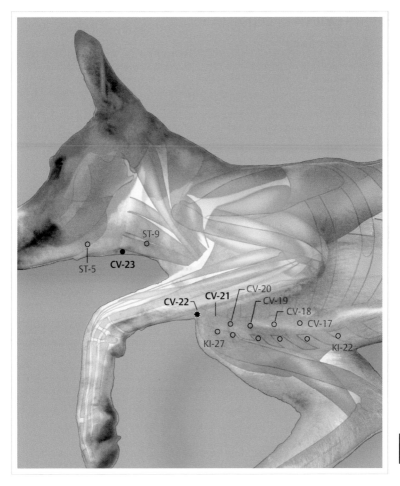

CV-24 Sauce Receptacle

承浆 *Cheng Jiang*

Intersection point with the governing vessel (*du mai*) and the large intestine and stomach channels.

Effect Dispels internal wind, supports the face, regulates the controlling vessel (*ren mai*).

Indications Facial nerve paresis, stomatitis, toothache, hypersalivation, torticollis.

Localization In the middle of a groove between the lower lip and the chin.

Technique To a depth of about 0.3 cun; perpendicular insertion.

CV

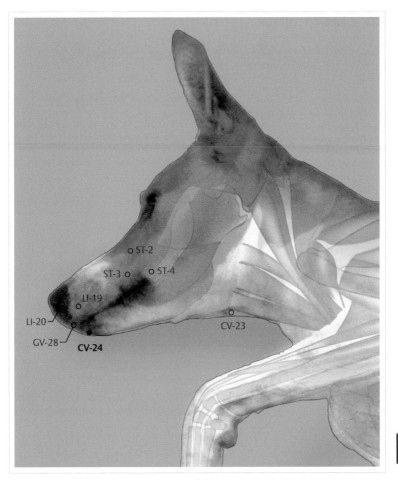

25 Extra Points

This chapter presents a selection of classic points for small animal acupuncture with special localization and effect as well as more recently discovered effective points outside the general channel courses or point localizations, which are partly analogous to points in humans. The points described here have proven their value in small animal practice.

The following points can be found in different sources with information varying from source to source. Wherever possible, alphanumeric identifications have been added.

Peaceful Spirit
安神 *An Shen*

Effect Calms the *shen*.

Indications Deafness, otitis.

Localization Caudal to the base of the ear, halfway between GB-20 and TB-17.

Technique To a depth of about 0.3 cun; oblique insertion in the direction of the contralateral eye.

Tip of the Ear
耳尖 *Er Jian*

Effect Draws out wind-heat.

Indications Shock, heat stroke, high fever, otitis, eye diseases, colic.

Localization On the convex tip of the auricle.

Technique To a depth of about 0.2 cun; perpendicular insertion; for best effect, let it bleed.

Kai Zhin Jui

Effect Moves *qi* stagnation.

Indications Mobilizes the iliosacral joint.

Localization On the lateral edge of the temporal muscle between the mandibular joint and the anterior edge of the base of the ear.

Technique To a depth of about 0.5 cun; oblique insertion in a rostral direction.

EX

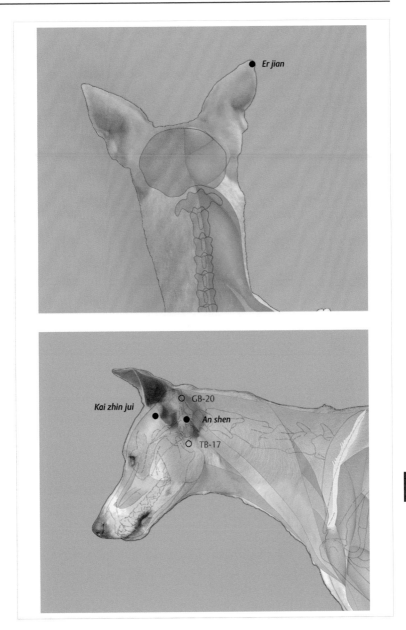

Track on the Forehead

Yin Tang

Effect   Supports the nose and eyes.

Indications   Frontal sinusitis, rhinitis, allergy, nasal congestion, eye pain, dizziness with nausea.

Localization   On the midline on the head between the two canthi of the eyes.

Technique   To a depth of about 0.3 cun; perpendicular insertion.

Great *Yang*

Tai Yang

Effect   Supports the head and eyes.

Indications   Facial nerve paresis, headache, eye problems.

Localization   In a depression of the temple, above the superficial temporal vein, about 1 cun behind the outer canthus of the eye.

Technique   To a depth of about 0.2 cun; tangential insertion.

EX

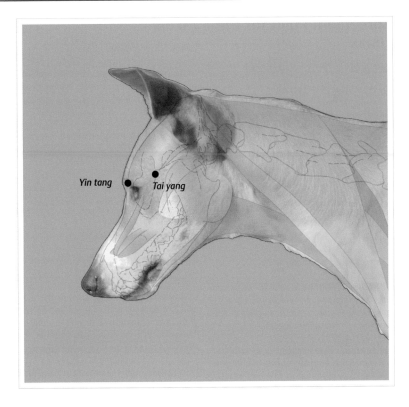

Agreement Point for the Elbow

Zhou Yu

Effect Moves *qi* stagnation.

Indications Elbow pain, elbow arthritis, paralysis of the foreleg.

Localization Between the lateral epicondyle of the humerus and the olecranon.

Technique To a depth of about 0.2 cun; perpendicular insertion.

Ling Ku

Effect Regulates and moves *qi*.

Indications Prostatitis, painful urination, used in combination with *da bai* for sciatica, stabbing pain along the outside of the hind leg, use contralateral point.

Localization Between the first and second toe on the forepaw, on the large intestine channel, proximal to LI-4 and exactly distal to the beginning of the metacarpal bone.

Technique To a depth of about 0.3 cun; perpendicular insertion.

Da Bai

Effect Regulates and moves *qi*.

Indications High fever, used in combination with *ling ku* for sciatica, stabbing pain along the outside of the hind leg, use contralateral point.

Localization Between the first and second toe on the forepaw, on the large intestine channel, slightly distal to LI-4.

Technique To a depth of about 0.2 cun; perpendicular insertion.

Zhong Bai

Effect Moves *qi* stagnation, harmonizes the triple burner.

Indications Lower back pain in the area L2–L3, especially pain when standing up; used in combination with *ling ku* and *da bai* for sciatica; use contralateral point, for edemas of the extremities, bilaterally.

Localization Between the fourth and fifth metacarpal bones, in a depression proximal to the metacarpophalangeal joint, about 0.2 cun above TB-3.

Technique To a depth of about 0.2 cun; perpendicular insertion.

EX

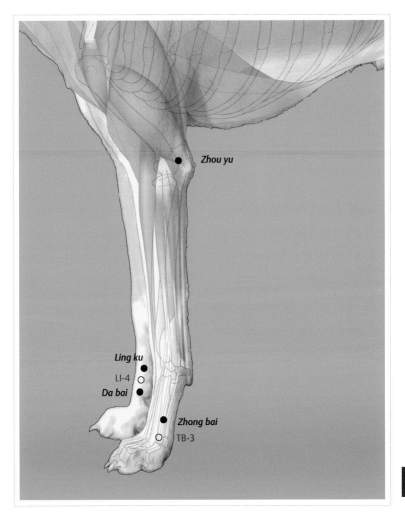

So Jing Dien

Effect Moves *qi* stagnation.

Indications Pain and stiffness in the back of the neck.

Localization On the forepaw between the third and fourth metacarpal bones, approximately at the level of TB-3.

Technique To a depth of about 0.2 cun; perpendicular insertion.

Chung Tze/Chung Hsien

Effect Moves *qi* stagnation.

Indications Pain in the back between the shoulder blades; needle both points together contralaterally.

Localization Palmar between the first and second toes about 0.2 cun above (*chung hsien*) and below (*chung tze*) LI-4.

Technique To a depth of about 0.2 cun; perpendicular insertion.

Anterior Interdigital Points

Ba Xie

Effect Moves *qi* stagnation, clears heat.

Indications Foreleg paralysis, contusions and sprains of the paw, gingivitis.

Localization Between the distal heads of the metacarpal joints on the forefoot.

Technique Insertion parallel to the toes from anterior through the toe web to a depth of about 0.4 cun; perpendicular insertion.

EX

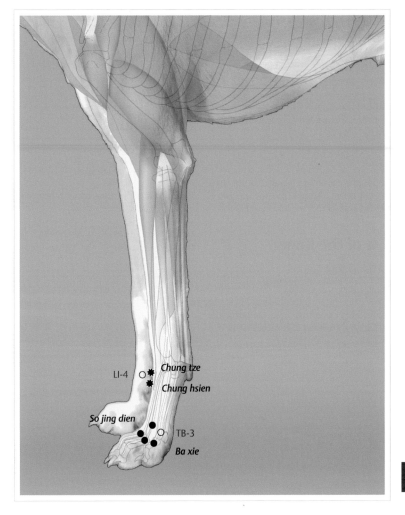

LI-4

Chung tze

Chung hsien

So jing dien

TB-3

Ba xie

Posterior Interdigital Points

Ba Feng

Effect   Moves *qi* stagnation, clears heat.

Indications   Hind leg paralysis, contusions and sprains of the paw, gingivitis.

Localization   Between the distal heads of the metacarpal joints on the hind foot.

Technique   Insertion parallel to the toes from anterior through the toe web to a depth of 0.4 cun; perpendicular insertion.

Eye of the Knee

膝眼 *Xi Yan*

Effect   Moves *qi* stagnation, clears heat.

Indications   Gonarthrosis, gonarthritis, strains and swelling in the knee joint.

Localization   Below the patella, bilaterally in the depression next to the straight patellar ligament; the lateral point is identical with ST-35.

Technique   To a depth of about 0.5 cun; perpendicular insertion.

Ovary Point

Nuancho

Effect   Moves stagnating *qi*.

Indications   Functional disorders of the ovaries, ovarian cysts.

Localization   Lateral to and below the transverse process of the fourth lumbar vertebra.

Technique   To a depth of about 0.3 cun; perpendicular insertion.

EX

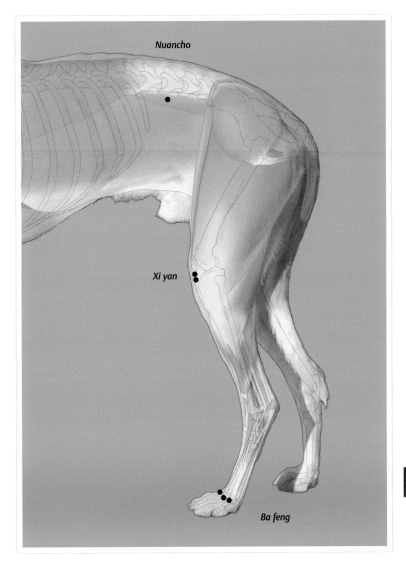

Nuancho

Xi yan

Ba feng

EX

Hua Tuo's **Paravertebral Points**

华陀夹脊 *Hua Tuo Jiaji*

Effect and Indications Has a segmentally supporting effect on the underlying organ.

Localization 0.5 cun lateral to each dorsal vertebra, between the governing vessel and the internal bladder channel.

Technique To a depth of about 0.3 cun; perpendicular insertion.

 Risk of pneumothorax in the area of the ribs.

Stop Bleeding

断血 *Duan Xue,* **Central One Also** *Tian Ping*

Effect Resolves blood stasis.

Indications All forms of hemorrhaging.

Localization Three points on the dorsal midline, one between the spinous processes of the thoracolumbar transition and one each in the front and back.

Technique To a depth of about 0.5 cun; perpendicular insertion.

Four Points

Si Liao

Effect Moves *qi* stagnation.

Indications Weakness of the hind leg, lower back pain, infertility, metritis.

Localization 0.5 cun lateral to the sacrum on both sides; there are four acupuncture points in a row: The first point is located in the first sacral foramen, the last point in the second sacral foramen, and the central points are located evenly spaced in between.

Technique To a depth of about 0.5 cun; perpendicular insertion.

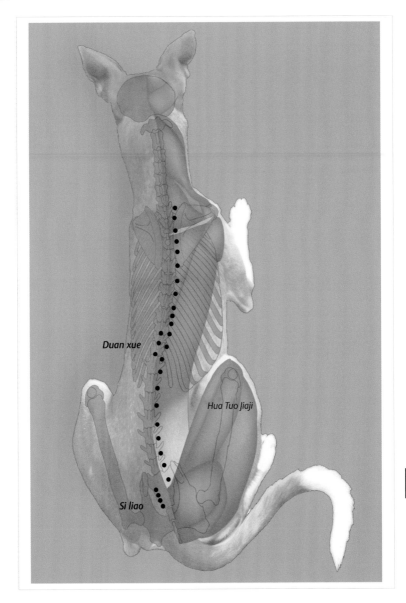

Duan xue

Hua Tuo Jiaji

Si liao

EX

Tip of the Tail

尾尖 *Wei Jian*

Effect Supports the lower spinal column and lumbar region, eliminates heat, moves *qi* stagnation.

Indications Paralysis of the tail or hind leg, cauda equina syndrome, colic, heat stroke, shock.

Localization Dorsally a short distance before the very tip of the tail.

Technique To a depth of about 0.2 cun; oblique insertion in a cranial direction.

Coccygeal Vertebra

Wei Jie

Effect Moves *qi* stagnation.

Indications Paralysis of the tail, weakness of the hind leg.

Localization On the dorsal midline of the tail, between the first and second coccygeal vertebrae.

Technique To a depth of about 0.2 cun; perpendicular insertion.

EX

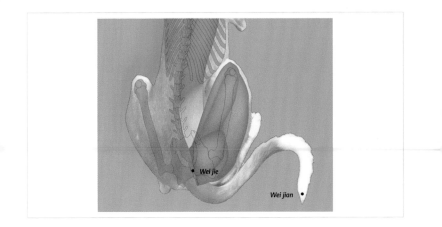

26 Subject Index

27 Points Index

Note: Page Numbers in *italics* refer to illustrations